SUSPICION

SUSPICION

VACCINES, HESITANCY, AND THE AFFECTIVE
POLITICS OF PROTECTION IN BARBADOS

Nicole Charles

Duke University Press   Durham and London   2022

Printed and bound by CPI Group (UK) Ltd, Croydon, CR0 4YY
Project editor: Lisa Lawley
Cover designed by A. Mattson Gallagher
Text designed by Aimee C. Harrison
Typeset in Garamond Premier Pro by Copperline Book Services

Library of Congress Cataloging-in-Publication Data
Names: Charles, Nicole, [date]- author.
Title: Suspicion : vaccines, hesitancy, and the affective politics of
protection in Barbados / Nicole Charles.
Description: Durham : Duke University Press, 2022. | Includes
bibliographical references and index.
Identifiers: LCCN 2021013191 (print)
LCCN 2021013192 (ebook)
ISBN 9781478015017 (hardcover)
ISBN 9781478017639 (paperback)
ISBN 9781478022251 (ebook)
Subjects: LCSH: Papillomavirus vaccines—Social aspects—Barbados. |
Papillomavirus vaccines—Political aspects—Barbados. | Health and race—
Barbados. | Biopolitics—Barbados. | Women, Black—Medical care—
Barbados. | Cervix uteri—Cancer—Barbados—Prevention. | Feminist
theory—Barbados. | BISAC: SOCIAL SCIENCE / Gender Studies |
MEDICAL / Infectious Diseases
Classification: LCC QR189.5.P36 C437 2021 (print)
LCC QR189.5.P36 (ebook) | DDC 616.9/11—dc23
LC record available at https://lccn.loc.gov/2021013191
LC ebook record available at https://lccn.loc.gov/2021013192

Cover art: Simone Asia, *Waterlogged*, 2015. Pen and ink on paper.
Courtesy of the artist.

Publication of this book is supported by Duke University Press's
Scholars of Color First Book Fund.

For my ancestors
and my matriarch,
Monica Marianne Charles

Contents

Acknowledgments

The first version of this manuscript took shape during my time in graduate school at the Women and Gender Studies Institute (WGSI) at the University of Toronto, where I began my scholarly engagement with transnational feminist studies. I am forever grateful to have been among M. Jacqui Alexander's final cohort of students at the WGSI. Thank you, Jacqui, for modeling transnational feminist activism in your teaching and scholarship, for reminding me that the archive is alive, for asking the most urgent and challenging questions, and for your persistent reminder "to take it there," to the roots, residues, and depths of any inquiry, to the feelings this digging unearthed, and to those who dig/dug alongside me. I also benefited immensely from the support of my extraordinary dissertation co-supervisors, now colleagues, Michelle Murphy and D. Alissa Trotz, who have guided this project from its infancy. Murphy, your confidence in me and excitement about this work have sustained me, and I am a better thinker because of you. Alissa, what a brilliant and generous force you are. Thank you for investing in me and for your endurance. I am deeply grateful to have met and been mentored by you.

I have had many wonderful opportunities to present and receive meaningful questions and feedback on portions of this work across several National Women's Studies Association conferences, Caribbean Studies Association conferences, American Studies Association conferences, Society for Social Studies of Science conferences, and invited talks at the Women's Studies and Feminist Research Speaker Series at Western University, the Feminist Lunch Series at the University of Toronto Mississauga, the Institute of Gender and Development Studies: Nita Barrow Unit at the University of the West Indies (Cave Hill, Barbados), and the Women's, Gender and Sexuality Studies Program at Barnard

College. Many thanks to the organizers of these events and to those in attendance who thoughtfully engaged with my work. Sections of the introduction, chapter 1, and chapter 3 appeared in an earlier form in an article in *Feminist Formations*, and an earlier version of chapter 2 appeared in an article in *Social Text*.

Thank you to Courtney Berger at Duke University Press for your investment in this book's possibilities, your guidance, and persistent enthusiasm from the beginning to the end. Thank you also to Sandra Korn and Lisa Lawley for guiding me through the production process. To my manuscript's two anonymous reviewers: what an honor it is to be read with such generosity. Thank you for the care with which you engaged with this book and the detailed and generative feedback you offered twice over.

I am indebted to all the Barbadian parents and teenagers who shared their stories with me over the many years of research for this book and who allowed me to journey with them through the intricacies of suspicion. I am thankful for the support of the Barbados Ministry of Health and the many public health professionals who provided me with a deeper understanding of the sociomedical and political landscape in Barbados from which I could begin to understand human papilloma virus (HPV) vaccination delivery. Thank you to the many incredible Caribbean feminist scholars who have read alongside me and supported the research and writing of this book during my time in Barbados, with special thanks to Peggy Antrobus, Charmaine Crawford, Tonya Haynes, and Halimah De Shong.

At the University of Toronto, I have had the great fortune to learn from and alongside Nikoli Attai, Sonny Dhoot, Cornel Grey, Zoë Gross, Brianna Hersey, Casey Mecija, and Henar Perales.

R. Cassandra Lord, it has been such a gift to have you as a colleague and dear friend. Thank you for bearing witness to it all and for helping me "keep it moving." Thank you, Dina Georgis, for serving on my dissertation committee, for pushing me to think more about the affective residues of suspicion, and for your gentle encouragement along the way. My colleagues W. Chris Johnson, June Larkin, Marieme Lo, Melanie Newton, Karyn Recollet, Joanne Saliba, Judith Taylor, S. Trimble, and Lisa Yoneyama have also offered me invaluable encouragement, inspiration, and comfort on this journey. I am also thankful for the graduate students with whom I have had the great privilege of thinking and working at the WGSI. The Technoscience Research Unit and the McLuhan Centre for Culture and Technology at the University of Toronto have provided much-needed intellectual support and space to think collectively throughout this project. Thank you to Kristen Bos, Patrick Keilty, Kira Lussier, Natasha Myers, and Sarah Sharma, whom I have been lucky enough to be in conversation with in these spaces. Great thanks to Elizabeth Parke for convening a series of writing groups through the Collaborative Digital Research Space at the University of Toronto Mississauga and to those who showed up week after week. You have all supported me during the difficult final leg of this journey.

Thank you to the many other colleagues, friends, and scholars across countries and interdisciplinary academic fields who have thoughtfully engaged me and this book's many threads, ideas, and iterations over the years: Gulzar Charania, Carolyn Cooper, Kelly Fritsch, Anna Harris, Hiʻilei Hobart, Kamala Kempadoo, Susan Knabe, Tamara Kneese, Ruthann Lee, Julie MacArthur, Bonnie McElhinny, Anne McGuire, Heather Paxson, Jessica Polzer, Joan Simalchik, Christy Spackman, Luke Stark, Rinaldo Walcott, Ian Whitmarsh, and Rebecca Wittmann. To my sisters in the Black Feminist Health Science Collective, especially Moya Bailey, OmiSoore Dryden, Ugo Edu, and Sandra Harvey, your words and scholarship have been guiding forces in this project.

To my Trini-Toronto posse, past and present, who have celebrated the big and small milestones of my (life) journey: Erica Beatson, Mikey Clarke, Danielle Kandel Lieberman, Prem Khatri, Demetra Koutroumbas, Becky Mak, Renee Ouditt, Yannique Ragbeer, Mampuru Stollmeyer, and Ike Werner, thank you for nurturing me with your company, food, laughter, and friendship.

Thanks to my parents, Michelle and Brian Charles. Mum, it was you who insisted I first research the HPV vaccine years ago. Thank you for empowering me to seek answers to the questions I cared about. Dad, writing this book brought me closer to you. Thank you for hosting me throughout the research process and for your enthusiasm, humor, and love. My sister has shared in my every sadness and joy. Amara, our sisterhood is such a source of truth, pleasure, and sustenance in this world. Thank you for your exuberance, vulnerability, and dance moves. Finally, to Tristan: thank you for holding me up every day, in every way possible throughout the research and writing of this book. Thank you for listening to every story before it was written, for reading the many drafts, and for your openness to learning and growing with me through this project and in this life. My greatest love and appreciation are reserved for you.

SUSPICION

An Introduction

As I waited to meet with an immunization nurse one afternoon in January 2016, I sat in a quiet waiting room in an otherwise hectic Barbadian public clinic. "I'll be right with you," Nurse Dobbs yelled as she rushed past me for the third time, busy completing her immunization rounds. Painted on one of the clinic's walls was a vibrant pink and blue mural featuring a smiling Mickey Mouse hovering above a bright yellow door that led to an immunization room. Framing the door was a dilapidated sign that read "Immunizations," and a louvered window with multicolored seashell curtains flanked its left side. To the right of the door was what appeared to be an official, nonlocal public health poster detailing "How to hold a baby while breastfeeding," along with three corresponding images of a white woman nursing a newborn baby. But it was the single piece of paper casually affixed to the top of the yellow door with tape and a red thumbtack that most caught my attention. On the paper was printed a low-quality photograph of a young Black boy of about three or four years old, arms crossed, his striped shirt worn and dirty (figures I.1 and I.2). In contrast to many global public health adverts that feature haunting images of emaciated African children, in this image the boy's cheeks are full and he is wearing an animated facial expression complete with a side-eyed look, recoiling ever so slightly from a laughing, well-dressed woman who appears to be a tourist. Although we have only a glimpse of this woman's profile, the boy's face is in full focus—his mature expression offering us a sense of his indivudalism that invokes not pity but

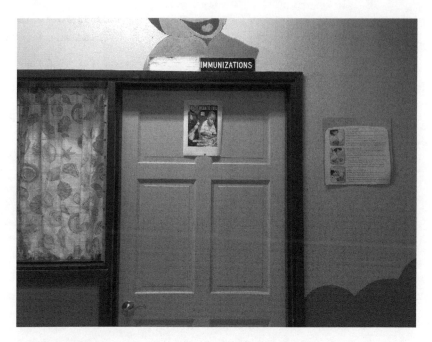

FIGURE 1.1 Polyclinic immunization waiting room in Warrens, Barbados, 2016. Photograph by the author.

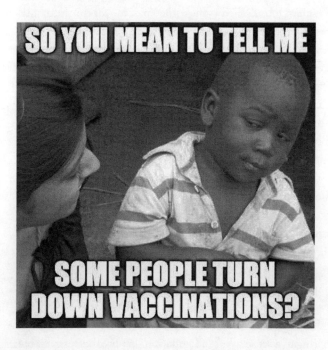

FIGURE 1.2 "Skeptical Third World Kid" meme. Reddit, June 20, 2012. www.reddit.com/r/pics /comments/vc0c9 /make_this _skeptical_kid _into_a_meme _stat_took/. Screenshot by author.

amusement. Text superimposed onto the image to correspond with the child's skeptical expression reads, "SO YOU MEAN TO TELL ME SOME PEOPLE TURN DOWN VACCINATIONS?"

The original photograph, taken in June 2012 in Gulu, Uganda, captures a still-unknown African child staring warily at an American doctor by the name of Heena Pranav who was visiting Uganda on a medical volunteer mission. Posted shortly thereafter to the social media and news aggregation website Reddit, a user on the platform implores others to "make this skeptical kid into a meme, STAT!"[1] Thereafter referred to as "Skeptical Third World Kid" online, this photograph went on to become a viral sensation. Copied and captioned with various phrases, the image grew to become the site of popular memes that juxtapose supposedly irrational Western behaviors, actions, and attitudes with the skepticism expressed by this young Ugandan child.

Not only do such memes perpetuate the narrative of Africans in need of humanitarian aid and salvation from the West, but as they proliferate behind digital screens as popular culture commodities in the West, they invite recognition, laughter, and perhaps pleasure in the trivial nature of "First World" problems as reflected in the cynical expression of this boy.

This particular meme, attached to the door of the immunization room, notably trivializes vaccine refusal. It suggests that those who might decline immunizations are less informed, knowledgeable, or educated than even the young boy in this image, who would seemingly always accept vaccinations, without hesitation, if only he were given the chance. Alongside the text that expresses the boy's bewilderment over the decision to decline vaccinations, his facial expression and posturing insinuate a simultaneous disbelief and disappointment in this choice despite and amid the immense privilege that often accompanies living in places like the United States. Together, his incredulous stare and these trenchant words suggest not merely a critique of vaccination refusal but the boy's gratitude for the medical care and services provided by US doctors such as Pranav, and the opportunities she affords to him and others in need.

Unsettled, I worried about this meme's suggestion that those who were ambivalent about vaccines were ungrateful, perhaps indifferent to the medical benevolence of those who make vaccines readily available in Barbados, in light of their shortage in places like Uganda. I wondered, Why post this image here, in this clinic? In placing this meme in a government-funded medical facility, was Barbados to be positioned in contrast to places like Uganda and places outside the developing world? Were Barbadians meant to smirk, to recognize themselves as privileged, educated people who ought to know better, be better than skeptical, hesitant, or resistant to vaccines? What does it actually mean to be vaccine "hesitant," as is commonly claimed by medical professionals in reference to people who express ambivalence toward vaccines? How does hesitancy relate to skepticism? What are we to make of vaccine hesitancy in postcolonial Barbados? As an already suspiciously perceived Trinidadian in Barbados with whom many medical professionals would cautiously speak if only because of the potential for my research to assist their quest to improve vaccine compliance, I dared not ask these questions to the nurse I was about to interview. *Suspicion* wrestles with these thorny questions as a means of complicating the biomedical conception of vaccine hesitancy and unsettling the plethora of misunderstandings, stereotypes, and injurious histories that undergird medical claims to hesitancy around the HPV vaccine in relationship to young women in Barbados—many of which are invoked in this meme.

HPV and Vaccine Hesitancy

HPV is a species-specific DNA virus that infects epithelial cells of the human body, including those of the fingers, hands, mouth, anus, vagina, esophagus, and cervix. With more than 150 different strains, HPV is the most common sexually transmitted disease worldwide, and it is estimated that more than 80 percent of sexually active women and men will encounter a sexually transmitted HPV infection in their lives.[2] While most HPV infections are asymptomatic and clear without treatment, persistent infection with high-risk strains of HPV can develop into precancerous lesions, cervical cancer, head and neck cancers, and genital cancers, including cancer of the anus, vulva, penis, and vagina.[3] The Caribbean is currently among the top four subregions in the world with respect to the incidence of cervical cancer and has the highest burden of HPV in the Americas.[4] In Barbados specifically, cervical cancer is the third most common female cancer in women ages fifteen to forty-four years, and it is estimated that 38 new cervical cancer cases are diagnosed annually in a population of under 300,000.[5]

In light of this high incidence rate and the promise of a vaccine to target the human papillomavirus, Barbadians' initially low uptake of the HPV vaccine came as a surprise to many local medical practitioners. Yet (HPV) vaccination hesitancy is not without historical and international precedent. Cultural and political anxieties around the safety, efficacy, and legitimacy of inoculation practices including variolation and vaccination are as old as vaccines themselves.[6] Since at least 2014, there has been a marked increase in cases of measles around the world, growing rates of polio outbreaks in sub-Saharan Africa and the Middle East, and a resurgence of whooping cough and mumps in the United States, Australia, and the United Kingdom.[7] The recent development and distribution of new cancer vaccines such as the HPV immunization, which protects against cervical and other HPV-related cancers, has presented governments with a host of new challenges surrounding vaccine compliance in adolescent and adult populations. Understanding vaccine hesitancy—a phenomenon defined by the World Health Organization (WHO) as the delay in acceptance or complete refusal of vaccines—has become an urgent international public health priority.[8]

According to the WHO Strategic Advisory Group of Experts, those who are vaccine hesitant fall on a continuum between complete acceptance and refusal and should be diagnosed for the specific determinants of their hesitancy.[9] In this framework, hesitancy is viewed as "complex and context specific, varying across time, place and vaccines . . . [and] influenced by factors such as complacency, convenience and confidence."[10] Here, *complacency* is understood by public health and medical professionals as a perceived lack of need for or value placed on vaccines. *Convenience* refers to one's access to vaccines, and *confidence* speaks to the (dis)trust in vaccines or one's provider.[11] Apart from public knowledge deficits in the science of vaccines, hesitancy is also understood by public health professionals to be closely aligned with and influenced by a range economic, political, and sociocultural factors.[12] A growing body of social science research on vaccine hesitancy has similarly focused on deciphering its broad-ranging and complex determinants.[13] Comparative ethnographies on vaccine hesitancy across the developing world, for instance, compellingly highlight the complex, interrelated, and multifaceted nature of factors that can affect one's hesitancy, including history and politics, religion, mode of vaccine delivery, distrust of the pharmaceutical industry, and the broader health system in which particular vaccines are introduced.[14]

Despite the recognition of hesitancy's complexity across these divergent bodies of literature, popular science texts and news media often conflate the phenomenon and those who identify as vaccine hesitant with antivaccination views.[15] Although vaccine hesitancy might entangle with antivaccine sentiment for some citizens in specific locations, as a phenomenon, it is not subsumable to it. To suggest so overlooks hesitancy's multiple constitutive factors, risks failing to address them (and thus the biomedical problem that is hesitancy in public health efforts to increase vaccine compliance), and, for my interests here, discursively misconstrues hesitancy as just a delay or refusal purportedly rooted in ignorance. Intervening in the bourgeoning landscape of social science and humanities research on vaccine hesitancy research, this book wrestles with the term *hesitancy* in relationship to the HPV vaccine by looking to how Afro-Barbadians vernacularly reframe this scientific terminology through the language of suspicion.[16]

Suspicion, this book asserts, is the affective intensity that Afro-Barbadians attach to the HPV vaccine around the lives and bodies of young Barbadian women, amid and alongside a range of bourgeoning bio- and information technologies in contemporary Barbados. Suspicion foregrounds Afro-Barbadians' gut feelings, emotions, and colonial residues of trauma from biopolitical harms and engenders forms of skepticism through which they often inconceivably reason to protect their children by refusing potentially life-saving technologies such as the HPV vaccine. In spite of the potentially fraught implications for the health of Barbadians, this book illustrates that suspicious affects indirectly reveal the complexity of the scientific logics and knowledge-making implications around refusal, protection, and care and promise capacious insights for the parents who stay true to their embodied sensibilities and for medical practitioners, feminists, and transnational, (techno)science, and humanities scholars, themselves hesitant to produce conceptually neat end points to inescapably entangled biopolitics of past and present.

The contemporary language of vaccine hesitancy and its preclusions can be situated in the lineage of medical discourse on noncompliance, which emerged in the United States in the 1950s in response to patients' resistance or incapacity to abide by biomedical prescriptions. Established as both an ideology of social control and a popular research subject in medical literature by the 1970s, the term *noncompliance* developed from "a continuity of prior patient-categories such as the 'recalcitrant', the 'careless', and the 'defaulter.'"[17] Though the word functioned to bolster physicians' sense of authority, it received repeated criticism by both lay and academic audiences for its underlying assumptions of patient passivity, ignorance, and blind submission to the authority of medical providers, and by the mid-1990s it was replaced by medical professionals with the less authoritarian term *nonadherence*.[18] Although the term was intended to foreground the role of patients as active participants in their health care decision making, medical anthropologists have reiterated how *nonadherence* similarly places the responsibility for drug uptake and efficacy on patients, rather than precarious health care structures and medical systems.[19]

Medical anthropologist Ian Whitmarsh has traced how discourses of noncompliance and nonadherence in Barbados have been widely adopted by doctors, pharmaceutical companies, and public health and nongovernmental institutions alike to explain high levels of asthma in the country. Conflating citizens' improper use of inhalers with a culture of irrationality and fearfulness in Barbados, he argues, both the language and ideology of noncompliance preclude attention to the risk factors associated with pharmaceutical products and the skepticism toward the medicalization of care that inheres with Barbadians' medical decision making and pharmaceutical consumption.[20] Rather than indicating ignorance or fear, Whitmarsh suggests, Barbadians' improper use or hoarding of unused medications might reveal citizens' widespread frustrations and even critiques of the Barbadian government's embrace of a culture of biomedicine focused on pharmaceuticals. In this context, Barbadians' so-called cultural failure to comply makes precarious the very category of medical compliance and its construction of rationality.

Appearing most prominently in medical literature since 2011, the phrase *vaccine hesitancy*, like nonadherence and noncompliance, fails to capture the multiple affects and experiences involved in vaccination decision making, which often transcend the individual and the contemporary.[21] Terms such as *hesitancy*, like the "Skeptical Third World Kid" meme, participate in a culture of biomedicine that is often frustratingly inattentive to the weight history continues to bear on peoples of African descent as they encounter and navigate the institution of medicine and its plethora of new biotechnologies. Elaborating Whitmarsh's questioning of nonadherence and noncompliance frames in Barbados in new ways, *Suspicion* unsettles the term and sedimented biomedical logics of hesitancy and furthermore insists on the historical significance, contemporary relevance, and fraught and generative nature of the presumed unsettling nature of Afro-Barbadians' suspicion.

In characterizing hesitancy as unsettling, public health and medical practitioners adopt the word to indicate worry and concern, not simply around the implications of vaccine hesitancy for the spread of diseases but around the risk they believe hesitancy and public distrust threatens to impose on modern democratic societies. Much of what is unsettling about vaccine hesitancy, this book argues, is the extent to which it contests the hegemony of uncontested scientific and biomedical certainty and truth. Critical feminist, technoscience, Black, Indigenous, queer studies, and decolonial scholars have often characterized their work as engaged in a politics of troubling and unsettling, referring to unsettling here as that which agitates, makes anew, and makes unstable such hitherto uncontestable claims to knowing and being. Black studies and Black queer diaspora scholarship has consistently engaged in unsettling the nation-state, reconfiguring its boundaries, and destabilizing Black heteropatriarchy.[22] Indigenous feminist and decolonial theorists have explicitly deployed the term *unsettling* in different ways to disrupt the ongoing process of settler colonialism, unsettle the lands that have been "settled," and critically embrace the agitation, worry, discomfort, and sense of unsettlement that emerges for white settlers through this politic.[23] Likewise, sticking and reckoning with these troublesome affects, feminist technoscience scholars have variously embraced fraught and contestable matters of care, piracy, and our relations to the Earth.[24] Following these moves to unsettle, *Suspicion* reveals both what is unsettling and what is dismissed in the designation of Barbadian parents as lying hesitantly on a spectrum, in need of advice and reassurance to assist them in improving and sustaining vaccine confidence and reaching the end goal of acceptance of HPV immunization. This book argues for the usefulness of suspicion for those ambivalent about vaccines and for critical feminist, social science, and technoscience studies scholars wishing to attend simultaneously to colonial modes of scientific knowledge and contentious refusals of biomedicine in the anglophone Caribbean—a region that is witness to increasing access to biotechnologies like vaccines and existing in the wake of neoliberal globalization, rapid socioeconomic and technological changes, and violent colonial regimes in which coercive biomedical techniques have long necessitated suspicion and alarm from colonized peoples.[25]

As *Suspicion* details, Barbadian parents' biomedically prescribed irrationality or hesitancy toward the HPV vaccine fails to account for these multiple and complex historical, transnational realities. By vernacularly reframing hesitancy as suspicion, I argue, Afro-Barbadians offer a thickened articulation of these multilayered and palimpsestic memories, realities, and contexts as affective intensities that, while location-specific, hold transnational implications. *Suspicion* emphasizes the continued salience of histories of persistent colonialism-capitalism in the anglophone Caribbean, of which science and medicine were and are an integral part. Suspicion demands that we sit in proximity to these histories. It implores that we rethink and revise our relationality to biomedicine, its inescapable entanglements in these histories of racism, pain, and discomfort and in the understandings of care that these pasts continue to animate across space and time. In the lineage of transnational Black feminist thought that finds the rubric of refusal for thinking and rethinking everyday vocabularies and practices of struggle against anti-Blackness to be urgent, *Suspicion* refuses the discourse and the unsettling genealogy of hesitancy and instead embraces the radical possibilities of suspicion as affect.[26] It thinks with and about suspicion and its excesses that circulate around and beyond the HPV vaccine in postcolonial Barbados. Moving from a discussion of suspicion's contemporary socioeconomic manifestations and historic circulations to an analysis of its fraught association with cultural tropes of respectability, hypersexuality, and protection in relation to Black women and Black female sexuality, this book tells a story of suspicion, its generativity and protective qualities, its impact on subject formation and transnational alliances, its relationship to certainty, and its inescapable fallibility.

The setting of this unfolding and circulating suspicion is postcolonial Barbados, which was under British control from 1627 to 1966, when it gained independence.[27] Barbados is the easternmost Caribbean country, stretching thirty-four kilometers in length and, according to locals, is just "a smile" wide. The populace consists primarily of Black nationals, the majority of whom are descendants of enslaved Africans. With a population of 286,641 as of 2018, Barbados is one of the most densely populated countries in the world.[28] Known for its well-developed education system and high standard of education, the country has also enjoyed one of the highest literacy rates in the world.

Unlike its mountainous and volcanic neighbors, Barbados has flat and undulating lands that historically contributed to the success of sugarcane as the most profitable crop from the colonial era through the early 1980s. After the mid-1980s saw a global decline in sugarcane prices and a move toward privatization and liberalization, manufacturing industries were no longer profitable for Barbados, leading the government to begin to promote foreign investment in tourism and provide tax incentives to the population to encourage manufacturing in the postindependence era.[29] Tourism and international business have since made up the major sectors responsible for the country's gross domestic product.[30]

The early formation of a two-party system (the Barbados Labor Party [BLP] and the Democratic Labour Party [DLP])—a cabinet government modeled on the British Westminster system—along with a sound economy, prepared Barbados for a smooth transition to independence in 1966 after more than three hundred years of colonization. Unlike other British Caribbean islands (such as Jamaica and Guyana), where the state played a dominant role in economic development after independence, the BLP and the DLP (who describe themselves as socially democratic) have historically supported private enterprise, public infrastructure, and regional integrative initiatives. Following a period of recession in the early 1990s accompanied by high foreign debt payments and social and political disequilibrium, the government established its now renowned social partnership in lieu of devaluing its currency and implementing structural adjustment policies as suggested by the International Monetary Fund.[31] Although this blend of industry and government partnership has been foundational to the long-standing success of the country's national education and health care systems, its historically competitive economy and for decades the highest-ranking Human Development Index (HDI) in the Caribbean, a sustained recession on the heels of the 2008 global financial downturn has had a grave effect on Barbados's economic and sociopolitical conditions. For many Barbadians with whom I spoke between 2015 and early 2018, this recession and its ripple effects of public sector layoffs, rising crime rates, and government instability were instrumental in breeding a deep sense of distrust toward the former government. Even as the country began to emerge from this recession in 2014, during my first research trip to Barbados from late 2015 to early 2016, I witnessed an unmistakable sense of apathy toward the then-DLP government, which remained widely characterized in public commentary by economic recession and resource scarcity.[32] Indeed, the country's rapidly falling HDI ranking, increased unemployment, and a retreat of the state from tertiary education funding all suggest that the long-standing social partnership between the Barbadian state and society had been fundamentally upset.[33]

Apart from exploring suspicion around the HPV vaccine in connection to young Afro-Barbadian women, *Suspicion* is attentive to the ways affective communities and climates of suspicion exist alongside and in response to these forms of neoliberal governmentality and the changing economic climate in Barbados. As I argue in chapter 1, these dynamics of economic uncertainty, state retreat, and a growing sense of government distrust are crucial to contextualizing Afro-Barbadians' contemporary reception and deliberation of newly introduced government initiatives, policies, and products such as the HPV vaccine, which emerge through an assemblage of state-biomedical and multinational pharmaceutical efforts to encompass a biocitizenship project.[34] As I have argued elsewhere, such projects "rely on the coalescence of industry marketing, state recommendations, and self-governance, to facilitate the mobilization of certain ... individuals" (in the Barbadian case, at first young Barbadian women and their parents) "to protect their at-risk, pre-damaged biologies" by choosing HPV vaccination.[35]

With a health care system at the center of the multinational pharmaceutical industry in the eastern English-speaking Caribbean, Barbados was one of the first Caribbean countries to introduce the HPV vaccine through a national program in 2014.[36] Gardasil, a quadrivalent vaccine manufactured by pharmaceutical company Merck, was the first vaccine to be approved by the US Food and Drug Administration (FDA) in June 2006 for use in girls and women ages nine to twenty-six to target four strains of HPV (6, 11, 16, and 18) which account for approximately 70 percent of cervical cancer cases and 90 percent of anogenital warts cases in the United States.[37] Since 2006, the HPV Information Centre estimates that Gardasil has been licensed for use in over one hundred countries. Though still most widely colloquially understood to provide protection against the noncommunicable disease of cervical cancer in girls and women, Gardasil provides protection against the aforementioned strains of the sexually transmitted human papillomavirus, which can variously result in precancerous lesions; cervical cancer; head, neck and throat cancers; and genital cancers, including cancer of the anus, vulva, penis, and vagina. In turn, shortly after its introduction onto the US pharmaceutical landscape, the CDC moved to recommend the use of Gardasil in boys and men ages nine to twenty-six to specifically prevent anal cancer and anogenital warts. Following the launch of the vaccine across European countries, US states, Canadian provinces, Australia, and multiple Caribbean countries including Barbados, governments appear to have followed this initial offering of the vaccine to women exclusively.[38]

In Barbados, the HPV vaccine was introduced through a national school-based vaccination program in January 2014 for girls ages ten to twelve years old.[39] Unlike the traditional introduction of new vaccines by nurses through the island's public clinics (polyclinics), implementing the HPV vaccine involved an unusual and extensive period of public sensitization training, media broadcasts, flyers, town hall meetings, and parent-teacher association meetings run by a team of specially appointed immunization nurses to inform the Barbadian public of the availability and necessity of the vaccine. Through this new vaccination scheme, Ministry of Health immunization nurses would visit secondary schools to distribute parental consent forms for them to administer the vaccine to their daughters in subsequent school visits. Notwithstanding (in fact, possibly due to) these unexpected intensive promotional and sensitization efforts, local immunization nurses reported acceptance rates of a mere 19 percent at the end of 2014.[40]

In addition to a perceived resistance to the vaccine from parents, nurses lamented that many secondary school headmasters, guidance counselors, and teachers were similarly suspicious about the vaccine and the new mode of delivery, and speculated that teachers might have conveniently failed to distribute consent forms to students. These suspected actions, dismal uptake rates, the rise in public commentary, and concern over this new vaccine quickly indicated to medical professionals a growing prevalence of HPV vaccine hesitancy across the island in 2014.

Shortly after my arrival in Barbados in September 2015, the Ministry of Health changed its approach to delivering the vaccine in an attempt to circumvent what it felt was an overwhelming resistance. This change involved expanding the vaccination program to include secondary school girls under fifteen years of age in first, second, and third forms, and opening the vaccine to boys under fifteen years should their parents specially request it. To mitigate issues of resistance from teachers and guidance counselors, the ministry mailed consent forms to parents directly, but despite even these efforts, ministry officials noted that vaccine uptake rates remained unfavorable. By mid-2015, the Ministry of Health determined that the school-based immunization approach was ill suited to Barbados. It withdrew the vaccination program from schools and began administering the vaccine through the polyclinics. As of this writing, the primary recipients of the HPV vaccine are ten- and eleven-year-old primary school students. In an attempt to routinize the HPV vaccine, the ministry mandated that immunization nurses offer the vaccine to these students alongside diphtheria, tetanus, and polio booster shots, which they have traditionally received at polyclinics in preparation to enter secondary school.

Although many of the medical practitioners I spoke with over the course of my research argued that this new approach significantly minimized parents' hesitancy about the vaccine (as was evident, they argued, by the notable increases in vaccination uptake), both they and the parents I interviewed emphasized the continued and multiple suspicions that appeared to attach to the vaccine, the state, and the medicopharmaceutical assemblage behind the vaccine's introduction. In the moments such claims were uttered, I began to wonder about the potential differences between vaccine hesitancy and the term *suspicion*.

Theorizing Suspicion

It was only after Barbadian parents, nurses, and public health professionals used the word *suspicious* rather than *hesitant* to describe the feelings commonly associated with the vaccine that I came to investigate the politics of suspicion more fully. Like the term *hesitancy*, *suspicion* encompasses a sense of cautious reluctance and thought. But suspicion further denotes the act of suspecting, of apprehending guilt or fault, of feeling wary, uncertain, and distrustful. Like resistance, suspicion involves a sense of doubtfulness and withholding of certainty, but suspicion, this book asserts, ought not to be simplistically conflated with resistance or even refusal.

As a phenomenon, the term *resistance* has been widely theorized and critiqued across feminist and cultural anthropological scholarship.[41] The fields of anthropology and science and technology studies have seen a growing interest in theorizing the concept of refusal as a subject that is linked to but distinct from resistance for its productive social and political openings and ethical claims to the world. Embracing refusal's multiplicity, scholars have variously invoked the phenomenon as a capacious concept that surrounds and moves beyond the state and citizenship, a method evident within and in response to politics and political action, and a response to scientific advancements from reproductive technologies like amniocentesis to vaccines and stem cell transplants.[42] Tina Campt defines refusal as "the urgency of rethinking the time, space, and fundamental vocabulary of what constitutes politics, activism, and theory, as well as what it means to refuse the terms given to us to name these struggles."[43] As a Black feminist practice and commitment to reject the status quo that renders Blackness illegible, refusal simultaneously creates and names possibilities for recognition in the face of state-driven neglect and negation. Audra Simpson's *Mohawk Interruptus* similarly invites us to consider the generativity of refusal as both the everyday forms of interruption and disengagement that Indigenous peoples use and as an anthropological mode of inquiry that "acknowledges the asymmetrical power relations that inform the research and writing about native lives and politics" with an intention to honor and preserve tribal sovereignty and destabilize settler nationhood.[44] Building on Simpson's concept of ethnographic refusal, Kim TallBear emphasizes the "histories of privilege and denial" from which scientific and cultural understandings of biology and belonging increasingly emerge in the twenty-first century.[45] For TallBear, feminist and Indigenous refusals of these categories might be subsequently understood as the precipice of change from which new forms of technoscientific developments and cultural sovereignty can emerge for Indigenous peoples. Across scale and context, whether conceptualized as concept, subject, theory, or method, refusal must be recognized as significantly informed by "a complex interplay of [people's] past experiences (real and imagined), present circumstances, and future hopes and fears."[46] In conversation with this dynamic body of scholarship around refusal and Ruha Benjamin's caution against the "analytic summersaults" in which technoscience continues to engage to claim medical distrust as "inexplicable curiosit[ies]," *Suspicion* works to unsettle and depathologize vaccine hesitancy through the Barbadian framing of suspicion.[47]

Like refusal, suspicion is constitutive of and co-constituted by Afro-Barbadians' everyday histories, political realities, and researchers' (ethnographic) encounters and experiences in Barbados. Yet suspicion is not an active form of refusal. Instead, following my interlocutors, this book argues for suspicion as an embodied affective intensity. Rather than viewing suspicion as a practice, tactic, form of refusal, or mode of resistance to vaccination, this book locates suspicion as affective relation that circulates in the various socioeconomic, political, cultural, and historical formations that contextualize the vaccine, growing assemblages of multinational pharmaceutical networks and the state, and longer transnational histories of slavery, capitalist extraction, and public health. As I explore in chapter 1, although suspicion is often intentional, it is simultaneously affective because to experience suspicion is to be affected by the object with which one has contact. Building on and intervening in theories of affect and embodied epistemology situated in women of color and transnational feminisms, *Suspicion* explores the messy entanglements of health care work, biomedical authority, state priorities, and noninnocent histories of colonial medical injustice in Barbados to offer suspicion as a unique theoretical contribution to existing scholarship on affect and broader discussions in the Caribbean and beyond on the afterlives of slavery.

Since about 2000, scholars have increasingly begun to theorize affect according to a range of feminist, philosophical, and theoretical orientations.[48] Across these traditions, affect is variously theorized as sensational embodiments, motivations, and intensities that constitute relations and create social orders. The concept of affective economies, as usefully offered by Sara Ahmed, highlights how affects work by attaching themselves to bodies and spaces, mediating the relationship between them. These and other feminist theorizations of affect as capacities to feel that are sticky, contagious, physiological, and psychological importantly capture the ways emotions can shape us in unpredictable ways and diagnose material and social conditions.[49] In conceptualizing hesitancy as suspicion and suspicion as affect, it is insightful to conceive this emotional intensity as that which is sticky and contagious, circulating in affective economies that multiply and accumulate in value over time and space amid social, psychic, and material realms.[50]

Long before the so-called turn to affect, critical feminist theorists in the 1980s gestured to emotional intensities and embodied feelings of love, empathy, and care as crucial modes of knowledge to make sense of and resist oppressive social formations.[51] At the same time, Audre Lorde's and other queer, radical, and women of color deployments of eroticism, and what Gloria Anzaldúa and Cherríe Moraga refer to as "theor[ies] in the flesh," were foundational in introducing an understanding of affect and affective intensities as the modes through which women of color navigate survival and liberation.[52] These affective turns, Claudia Garcia-Rojas forcefully argues, are what destabilize much of the contemporary "White affects and White forms of knowledge" that have come to characterize the recognizable canon of affect theory today and that overwhelmingly disavow women of color feminisms.[53] Though not often labeled under affect studies, women of color feminist theory has long and fundamentally captured the affective intensities at stake for people of color and Third World women, enabling them to survive, more than survive, negotiate, and refuse the racialized and hegemonic systems that inhabit their lives. *Suspicion* extends this lineage of women of color and Black feminist scholarship that disrupts "White affect" studies, gesturing to the languages of the self through which Afro-Barbadians theorize their felt ambivalences and their enmeshment in matrices of (post)colonial violence, power, pain, and care.[54]

Along with these women of color feminist insights and political commitments to a language and politics of the self that are grounded in, on, and of the flesh, critical work in transnational feminist studies offers generative points of departure for exploring the submerged and entangled affective roots and processes in the Caribbean.[55] Specifically, transnational feminist theory provides a basis for understanding how affects such as suspicion are multiply layered, circulating across and between borders over time and bound up in and responsive to the sedimentation of conquest and colonialism.

Transnational feminist M. Jacqui Alexander analogizes the idea of the palimpsest to that of a parchment: "[One] that has been inscribed two or three times, the previous text having been imperfectly erased and remaining therefore still partly visible . . . The idea of the 'new' structured through the 'old' scrambled, palimpsestic character of time, both jettisons the truncated distance of linear time and dislodges the impulse for incommensurability, which the ideology of distance creates."[56] Arguing for a conception of modernity and matter as complexly layered, Alexander calls on us to rescramble our understandings of the "here and now," making the notion of time a question of itself.[57] To believe otherwise absolves new impetuses and iterations of history of their unsettling effects and falls prey to that "historical amnesia" Stuart Hall cautions against.[58] *Suspicion* mobilizes this analogy of the palimpsest as a metaphor to frame suspicion and identify how it shifts and intensifies through various itineraries across space, continuously attaching and reattaching itself to ideologies of science, rationality, nationalism, and capitalism in and across longer historical and political contexts of public health, race, and nationalism in Barbados and the anglophone Caribbean. Contributing to a body of transnational Black feminist scholarship attuned to the afterlives of slavery; the movement and mobilization of power, relationality, and affect across space and time; and the exacerbated inequalities produced by neoliberalism in the anglophone Caribbean and beyond, this book offers suspicion as both theory and praxis—as generative and fraught, sticky and contagious because it is palimpsestic, living and lasting in the body, in embodied memories and histories of Afro-Barbadians in ways that are difficult to let go. Moreover, this book argues, suspicion interrogates the biomedical offerings of care presented via the HPV vaccine. In so doing, I show, suspicion reveals care's inequalities and political stakes—by mapping how health care work, biomedical authority, state priorities, assemblages, and noninnocent histories of colonial medical injustice often unwittingly intertwine. Fraught as it is, this book highlights that suspicion ought to be not only something to be overcome but understood for its gestures toward less injurious forms of health care promotion.

Suspicion's empirical contributions further intervene across the interdisciplinary fields of science and technology studies, medical anthropology, and critical race studies, detailing Afro-Barbadians' responses to a critical public health campaign designated to ameliorate the high rates of cervical cancer. Indeed, despite the powerful advances vaccines promise to afford in places like Barbados and the wider Caribbean, *Suspicion* shows that many Afro-Barbadians' enthusiasm about the vaccine is hampered because of multifaceted concerns about widely theorized discourses and prescriptions of Black female sexuality in the Caribbean, the motivations of the pharmaceutical industry and its assemblages working to promote the vaccine, and the influx of new globalized technologies present in contemporary Barbados (of which the vaccine is one). Likewise, and as excerpts from Barbadian nurses and parents highlight, affects of suspicion hold the potential to shape citizens' engagements with technologies like the vaccine but also with biomedical, pharmaceutical, and governmental claims to certainty and knowledge about hesitancy, care, and protection. As suspicion attaches to the capitalist interests behind the pharmaceutical promotion of the vaccine and to tropes of hypersexuality and erotic subjugation under slavery, the term *hesitancy*'s "historical" tropes are revealed and situated in longer histories of racialized science, dispossession, and exploitation, all of which characterized the colonial period.

Undermining the three Cs of hesitancy (complacency, confidence, and convenience), suspicion, as articulated by Afro-Barbadian parents with whom I spoke, further highlights the tenuous and problematic nature not merely of hesitancy but of the HPV vaccine and its discursive, financial, and scientific logics. Positioned alongside predominant biomedical claims that vaccine hesitancy is an unsettling threat to public health, the integrity of vaccines, and modern democratic societies, an understanding of suspicion as a palimpsestic affect exposes and contests the legacies within which such claims lie. These are claims that in the Caribbean and much of the colonized world echo colonial imperatives to civilize and "save" physically and morally threatening Black colonial subjects through the logics of science. From eugenicist "scientific" beliefs of Afro-Caribbean people as uncivilized, lazy, barbarous, and responsible for the spread of tropical diseases and weakening of empire, to medical and legal forms of regulation implemented in response to colonial anxieties around the Black female body as a form of racial and sexual poison, often injurious and racialized forms of science and biomedicine were central to the project of colonialism.[59] Rather than emerging in resistance to vaccination, suspicion travels in time to intimately connect to these racialized histories and reaches forward to attach to devices like the HPV vaccine, to what many of the parents with whom I spoke deemed contemporarily ideologically proximate techniques and technologies of control. In complex ways and with variable implications for citizens' health, suspicion speaks back to and interrupts the claims to settled knowledge that biomedicine espouses through advocating for the vaccine as *the* means to care and protection. By situating suspicion toward this (bio)medical technology in Barbados in longer spatiotemporal, cultural, and political genealogies that animate contemporary suspicions toward state-led public health interventions, *Suspicion* challenges mainstream narratives of irrationality that undergird the discourses of hesitancy.

Methodological Frames

During my time in Barbados, I was witness to much speculation around the reasons for parents' hesitancy toward the HPV vaccine: from public health professionals' theories about parents' ignorance, miseducation, or distrust in science to the widespread lay and medical belief that it was a pervasive "cultural" concern around respectability, premature adolescent (female) sexuality, and the vaccine's relationship to sex that dissuaded many parents from accepting the vaccine for their teenage daughters. Rather than trying to determine the underlying factors behind Afro-Barbadians' concerns about the HPV vaccine, my research initially began with an interest in understanding how parents expressed their ambivalence to it and the effects of this "hesitancy" in Barbadian society. Working from the hypothesis that the phenomenon of vaccine hesitancy could be understood beyond nervous indecision, I wanted to know what was at stake, not only for Barbadian parents who were ambivalent about the HPV vaccine but for the adolescents to whom the vaccine was targeted and for the medical professionals who were onerously working to deliver the vaccine to the Barbadian public. How did they conceptualize and attempt to counter this hesitancy? How did adolescents view their parents' concerns? Were they aware of public commentary and perceptions about their bodies and their sexuality? How did medical professionals promote the HPV vaccine and counter vaccine hesitancy, and what public feelings did these actions engender? While this line of inquiry opened me to many of the histories that made up parents' hesitancy, it uniquely emphasized the affective nature of what I came to understand as *suspicion*, rather than hesitancy—less an active form of resistance toward something and more an embodied, affective, and felt response that circulates around the vaccine, its promotion, its purported risk management of adolescent female sexuality, and its complex entanglement in global biopolitical and state assemblages, past and present.

Though my fieldwork in Barbados began in 2015 by exploring these questions, I quickly came to investigate Afro-Barbadian parents' affective refusals and suspicions of the HPV vaccine. Over the course of eleven months between 2015 and 2018, my methodological approach to interviewing Barbadians about their experiences of suspicion was guided by a genealogically informed transnational feminist inquiry that attends to the local by tracing multiple lines of engagement elsewhere and at other times.[60] As a historical and relationally based feminist theory and analytic, transnational feminism foregrounds questions of race, conquest, sexuality, colonialism, and global capitalism while engaging with the theorizations of women of color feminists to generate understandings and critiques of social and cultural processes and their global imbrications across place, space, and time.[61] Throughout this book, I draw on transnational feminism as theory and methodology to map how suspicion is genealogically shaped and transformed by material, social, political, and economic forces internal and external to the Barbadian nation. Building on Alexander's aforementioned generative invocation of the palimpsest as an analogy for our complexly layered temporalities, I foreground the role of affective relations and formations such as suspicion amid the nonlinear movement of state technologies, techniques, global capital, and biopolitics in Barbados and the anglophone Caribbean.

In the tradition of transnational feminist work in and on the Caribbean, which has emphasized bringing into ideological proximity diverse geographical places and "historical" processes of colonialism with "modern" social formations and claims of nation-building, I not only ask why people experienced suspicion toward and around this vaccine but genealogically trace how suspicion emerges across time and place for differently situated Barbadians and in relationship to transnational contexts.[62]

My genealogical approach to this work began with reading secondary historical texts and accounts of colonial medicine, biopolitics, and reproductive health care in Barbados and the anglophone Caribbean. These histories, along with transnational feminist theorizations of the body politic, biopolitics, and temporality, were integral to my capturing of the entangled, cyclical histories and repertoires of suspicion toward biomedicine, public health, and discourses of risk in the history of the Caribbean.[63] I combined this historical analysis with in-depth interviews and informal discussions with parents, adolescents, and medical practitioners. Between 2015 and 2018, I conducted sixty in-depth interviews with middle-class, primarily Afro-Caribbean Barbadian adolescents, medical practitioners, and parents—most of whom had previously accepted all other childhood immunizations for their children but responded to my call, which specifically sought to interview parents who were ambivalent or hesitant about the HPV vaccine.[64] My recursive investigation also included media analysis of the vaccine's promotion and reception, which entailed analyzing Barbadians' commentary on the vaccine and its marketing via Facebook posts, newspaper editorials, and online discussion threads, and a discursive analysis of public health social media campaigns, flyers, memes, and print and online pharmaceutical advertising for the vaccine. Everyday conversation with Bajan friends and family members, participants at conferences at the University of the West Indies, and locals in weekend markets and cafés, as well as listening to radio talk shows and segments on the local TV station Caribbean Broadcasting Corporation and reading the prominent *Nation News* newspaper were also informative in this regard.[65]

Recruiting parents and teenagers was a painstaking and challenging task I came to attribute in part to the suspicion that attached toward me as a foreigner—specifically Trinidadian—researcher. Many of the parents I interviewed questioned why I was not doing this research in Trinidad, and others frequently assumed I was working on behalf of a pharmaceutical industry or medical establishment sent to persuade or coerce them into accepting the HPV vaccine because of my interest in their "hesitancy," my foreign status, and, as some noted, my affiliation with an international university.[66] Parents' suspicions toward me as a foreigner often meant they would not agree to talk to me unless they met me in person or I had been given the "all clear" by a friend or acquaintance I had previously interviewed. As such, I relied heavily on word of mouth, snowball sampling, and sharing my flyers on social media (primarily through Facebook) to connect with participants after having less success with posting flyers in public places like malls, local cafés, and coffee shops. This nonrandom sampling method, my use of social media, and the characteristics of the local venues where I posted my flyers meant I had less control over the subjects whom I interviewed. As a result, the distribution of parents and teenagers whom I had the opportunity to interview was confined to self-described, middle-class Afro-Barbadians.

Although there were evident variations in participants' levels of income and positionalities vis-à-vis the state, their overarching middle-class status meant that we met in their well-kept homes or local cafés, and more often than not, they drove their cars to meet me on the island's busy south coast. All of these parents, with the exception of two who were homemakers, held middle-upper-class jobs such as teachers, authors, office managers, sales representatives, hair stylists, business owners, consultants, and engineers. Throughout the book, I detail the various ways class was invoked by Afro-Barbadian parents and teen-agers in relation to suspicion. As were most Barbadians, the middle-class Afro-Barbadians I interviewed were offered the vaccine through the government's national vaccination program rather than through their doctors' clinics. As I detail within the book, although the HPV vaccine was available through select private doctors' offices, its prohibitive cost meant that only a few local physicians offered it privately. As such, and despite the limitations of the representativeness of my sample, the medical professionals and immunization nurses with whom I spoke confirmed the widespread prevalence of Barbadians' vaccine hesitancy across the island's demographics when the vaccine was initially introduced in 2014, as evidenced by low uptake rates, and their experiences speaking with parents at town hall and parent-teacher meetings.[67]

The medical professionals I interviewed included senior medical officers at the Ministry of Health, private pediatricians, general practitioners, gynecologists, and immunization nurses in the island's nine publicly funded polyclinics responsible for distributing the HPV vaccine through the national vaccine program. As the primary distributors of the vaccine to Barbadians across the socioeconomic spectrum, immunization nurses provided a unique and broad characterization of "vaccine-hesitant" Barbadian parents and their beliefs about their concerns, often across class.[68] Many of the health professionals I spoke with congratulated me on my research, noting the importance of its eventual findings for improving vaccine uptake. In retrospect, it appears that the reasons medical professionals appreciated my research and willingly participated in it are the same reasons many of the parents I interviewed were suspicious of it. Like doctors, many parents incorrectly assumed that the motivations behind my research were to increase vaccine compliance and were skeptical of me and my research on this account. Throughout this book, I engage with excerpts of my discussions with these doctors and nurses to provide their viewpoints on parents' suspicion and its underpinnings to better portray the medicopolitical landscape in Barbados and emphasize the differences in affective stances among differently constituted Barbadians.

The Chapters

The chapters that follow think with and about suspicion and its excesses around and beyond the HPV vaccine in Barbados. Moving from a discussion of suspicion's contemporary socioeconomic manifestations and historic circulation to an analysis of its fraught association with cultural tropes of respectability, hypersexuality, and protection, I tell the story of suspicion, its generativity, and its fallibility; its impact on subject formation and transnational alliances; its relationship to certainty; and its inescapable shortcomings.

Chapter 1, "Circles of Suspicion," introduces the book and provides an overview of how I came to follow suspicion as an affect that attached not only to the HPV vaccine but to non-Barbadian Caribbean citizens like myself and a range of biopolitical and economic policies, practices, and technologies introduced or supported by the Barbadian government. This chapter situates the socioeconomic environment into which the vaccine was introduced in Barbados to underscore the intensity with which suspicion is distributed spatially and suffused across the Barbadian state's seemingly banal political and economic maneuvers. By discussing the current culture of neoliberal globalization in Barbados through the country's membership in the Caribbean Community and Common Market, I trace the actualization of suspicion as it moves toward arrangements like this, its facilitation of intraregional migration, and related government policies and engagements that sought to promote economic growth and securitization in Barbados in the years immediately surrounding the 2014 introduction of the HPV vaccine. Detailing nurses' and parents' articulations of suspicion around the HPV vaccine, I highlight how suspicion similarly attaches to this biomedical technology in ways that are enmeshed in the economy but productive of relations and divides that transcend the economic realm.

Chapter 2, "Risk and Suspicion," explores how affects of suspicion have transitioned and intensified across time in Barbados and the anglophone Caribbean. Specifically, it situates suspicion around the HPV vaccine and its administration in Barbados in the long, racialized history of transatlantic slavery, its enmeshment in risk and capitalism, and its infrastructures of biopolitical surveillance. Tracing a particular set of instances within which risks to coloniality and postcoloniality have been managed through surveillance across time in Barbados and the British Caribbean from the 1780s to the present, this chapter highlights the imperative to study Black women as risk(y) and the role of biopolitics/biomedicine in mitigating these risks. Suspicion, this chapter shows, exists in a symbiotic relationship with the surveillance of risk and racialized biopolitics, attaching both to those holding these perceived risks and to the colonial officials and (post)colonial states attempting to mitigate these risks through racialized biopolitical techniques of care, control, and surveillance. In turn, this chapter illustrates how affects of suspicion materially and metaphorically recall colonial residues, prompting Afro-Barbadian parents to more closely interrogate pharmaceutical technologies like the vaccine and question the state's agenda in promoting them.

Chapter 3, "(Hyper)Sexuality, Respectability, and the Language of Suspicion," traces the contradictory articulations and theorizations of suspicion by adolescents, nurses, and parents as they relate to respectability politics, sex, and bio- and communication technologies in Barbados. Guided by adolescents' reflective commentary on the multiple silences and suspicions that surround their sexual bodies and technologies like the HPV vaccine, I begin by exploring how suspicion around the vaccine is understood by differently situated Barbadian citizens. In contrast to teenagers' and nurses' frequent claims that parents' suspicion toward the vaccine was indicative of a long-standing "cultural" concern about female hypersexuality and Afro-Caribbean peoples' subsequent adoption of a politics of respectability, Afro-Caribbean parents offered a more nuanced understanding of the ways respectability inheres in their concerns about state-led biomedical technologies. Reading parents' in-depth discussions of their suspicion in connection with feminist theorizations of respectability, I highlight how residues of suspicion reflect a complex navigation of hegemonic colonial stereotypes of Black female hypersexuality and a distrust of the postcolonial state and index a growing wariness of proliferating neoliberal global circuits of technoscience, ethics, economics, and pharmaceutical exchange of which this vaccine is a part. In the wake of a series of school sex scandals across the Caribbean from 2011 to 2016 in which cellphones were used to record teenagers' sexual activity, I broaden the discussion around suspicion to further review the language of suspicion as it attaches to communication technologies like smartphones and laptops and the adolescents who use them. Like the HPV vaccine, I argue, these technologies surface affects of suspicion, distrust, and anxiety for many Afro-Barbadian parents in relation to adolescent sex, often in unexpected ways.

In chapter 4, "Care, Embodiment, and Sensed Protection," I detail the multiple constitutions of sense and protection that the Barbadian doctors, nurses, and parents I interviewed variously forged around the HPV vaccine. Here I am especially interested in how Afro-Caribbean parents embody suspicion and frame these suspicions and subsequent refusals of the vaccine as ethical imperatives. Tracing the ethical encounters and narratives of protection these parents described to me, I argue that suspicion signals for these parents the limits of protection, reproduction, and futurity—categories that are especially complex in the "afterlife of slavery."[69] As something more than unsettling and problematic, suspicious affects and the modes of protection they engender are protective forms of self-determination and defense for Afro-Caribbean parents grappling with the sordid histories of those objects and policies to which suspicion attaches, histories that continue to inhabit the contemporary moment. These understandings of protection, I show, exist in opposition to the view of protection articulated by Barbadian medical professionals and the state in its biocitizenship struggle to introduce technologies like the HPV vaccine in the name of protection—importantly speaking back to injurious histories of care, yet holding potentially troubling implications for the health of Afro-Barbadian communities.

Chapter 5, "Suspicion and Certainty," pulls these lines of inquiry together to think more broadly about suspicion, its effect on subjectivity, and its existence amid the precarious projections of certainty espoused by the biomedical community. Although the doctors and nurses I interviewed were quick to attribute HPV vaccine hesitancy to antivaccination rhetoric online and the general ease with which unreliable medical information could be accessed, this chapter shows how suspicion continually exceeds even these boundaries, diffusing into the medical profession itself and existing alongside medical professionals' claims to certainty and truth around the HPV vaccine. Rather than viewing suspicion and certainty in an opposition, this chapter argues for a relational understanding of the two and illustrates the generative insights they offer public health practitioners and academics seeking to understand the racialized, gendered, historical, and affective politics of care and its presumed impediments. Situating parents' ideologies of suspicion, protection, and claims to self-determination in the context of Caribbean feminist and Afro-diasporic activism and advocacy around racialized communities' health from the 1970s to 1990s, the chapter ends with a consideration of the transformative potential certainty and suspicion collectively promise for improved public health promotion of HPV and its related diseases in Barbados.

ONE

Circles of Suspicion

One of the first calls I received in response to my recruitment flyers seeking "HPV-vaccine hesitant participants" was from Pamela, an Afro-Barbadian mother of two in her mid-forties. Pamela was excited to learn that I was affiliated with the University of Toronto and was interested in finding out more about my project. As I began to discuss my research, she abruptly asked, "[You] Trini?" Before I could fully respond, she continued, "I know so, [one] can't miss that accent," she said, chuckling. Speaking no more of it at the time, we continued on with our phone conversation to arrange an in-person interview. As I hung up, I thought more about my identity as a Trinidadian researcher and my naïve confidence before arriving in Barbados about the benefit my Trinidadian citizenship would offer in terms of interviewing locals despite my Canadian affiliation. Over the course of the first few weeks in Barbados, I continued to reflect on my positionality in fieldnotes, recognizing the multiple occasions on which I felt the need to reassure potential interviewees about my trustworthiness in response to a sensed unease or ambivalence about my motivations for conducting this research. Not only was I Trinidadian, I would stress, but Barbados was very much a second home to which I traveled frequently to visit relatives. Yet far from my Caribbean connections eliciting confidence and trust, I soon realized that my ascribed suspicion was partly due to my being Trinidadian, and I found myself embroiled in a daily negotiation of the tired and tiring insider/outsider researcher dilemma as I navigated what it meant to be deemed suspicious.

Most of the interviews I conducted with parents invariably began as they did with Pamela—opening with questions about my Trinidadian background (evident from my accent), and often concluding with a discussion of the then-unknown-to-me contentious relations many Bajans had with Trinidadians. My suspicious status, parents shared, was to do not only with my being Trinidadian but with the nature of my research, which some misconstrued as manipulative. To this end, I was often asked whether my "agenda" was the same as those of doctors and pharmaceutical companies interested in changing people's minds and increasing HPV vaccine compliance. In hopes of circumventing these particular concerns, making clear and at times defending my motivations for conducting this research, I occasionally and cautiously shared that my own Trinidadian mother was similarly ambivalent about the HPV vaccine when it was first approved by the Food and Drug Administration in the United States in 2006. In response to this disclosure, one mother, named Diane, smiled and said to me, "Okay, I see. But we don't call you Trinidadians you know, we call you Trickidadians. [You] come here and buy up all we banks and we supermarkets. Y'all is Trickidadians, man!" Here, in the same breath, she accepts my research and motivations as benign while reinforcing why I ought to be deemed suspicious. In this example, she references the momentous 2012 buy-out of the Barbados National Bank by the Trinidadian-owned Republic Bank Limited. While Republic Bank previously owned more than half the shares in Barbados National (64 percent as of 2010), its 2012 decision to acquire all remaining dissenting shares and become 100 percent owner was a painful moment for many Barbadians, who witnessed an effective replacement of their long-standing national bank.[1] Diane's comments further speak to what was then a more recent rebranding exercise conducted by the Trinidadian parent company, the Neal & Massy Group (now known as Massy Group) in 2014, during which Massy began rebranding several Barbadian supermarkets, convenience stores, pharmacies, distribution stores, and malls in an effort to strengthen its corporate identity. As another mother expressed to me, this rebranding served as final touches of a "Trinidadian takeover" in Barbados.

Despite my varied attempts to insert myself into particular affective relations with Barbadian parents in which suspicion about the vaccine could be openly shared, such statements reinforced that, by virtue of my Trinidadian identity, I should never be wholly trusted. While pointing out my otherness in such a facetious manner was indeed a form of affective relation, my attempt to draw on a range of positive affects that I assumed would naturally exist among fellow Caribbean citizens and the presumed-negative affects of suspicion to which my mother and many of the parents I interviewed were aligned failed to account for the complex economic and political dimensions involved in the way affects like suspicion circulate. Although often spoken in jest, comments like Diane's indexed the current Barbadian landscape, one that was inundated with intraregional and international corporations, interests, investments, researchers, and the like. While these interests often hold the potential to benefit the Barbadian economy (and are thus largely embraced by the Barbadian government), the psychic toll of the unwavering interest in Barbados and its assets on Barbadian people was palpable. The Barbadian government came under critique and suspicion by many of its citizens in this regard, both for complying with the multitude of intraregional acquisitions and overhauls that occurred through the early to mid-2000s under the Caribbean Single Market and Economy and for facilitating local initiatives and policies, which many suspect were actually implemented to comply with international principles. In this socioeconomic and political context, I came to understand suspicion—first in relationship to my positionality and subsequently as it connected and attached to the HPV vaccine.

Nurse Dobbs was one of the first immunization nurses I interviewed to discuss her experiences counseling parents who were hesitant toward the HPV vaccine. She began our interview by pointing to the word *suspicion* in relation to the vaccine. When I asked why parents had been so hesitant to give this vaccine to their children she responded, "Well, I don't know if it was fear or hesitancy. . . . I think it was . . . it was really just a lot of suspicion about the vaccine." This suspicion, she argued, arose from a complex assemblage of factors, including the vaccine's nontraditional rollout and marketing, and Barbadians' always already "suspicious" inclinations:

> Okay, take for example we've just had changes in the immunization schedule. There was no hurrah, there was no great output on the television about it. We told the parents we are introducing an injectable version of an old vaccine and, okay, fine. It was readily accepted; you know? Because there was no big fanfare. So, I think a lot of it had to do with the way we introduced the vaccine, and if you do something like that with a suspicious population at best (Barbadians are very secretive and [Barbados] is a close-knit society), so you do that and word gets out and this body is saying this and that body is saying that and, you know.[2]

Nurse Dobbs, like many others with whom I interacted, used the adjective *suspicious* to describe her patients' feelings toward the HPV vaccine, how it was introduced to the public, and her fellow citizens and Barbadian culture more generally. While I was well aware of the suspicion that attached to me, and was becoming increasingly attuned to its wider circulations in the political economy, prior to this conversation I had neither considered the word *suspicion* in relation to the HPV vaccine, nor did I appreciate how Barbadians invoked the word in relationship to the biomedical discourse of hesitancy. I became intrigued by this idea of suspicion, its relationship to the term *hesitancy*, and how Barbadians invoked the term to characterize their attachments and relations to the vaccine.

According to the *Oxford English Dictionary*, suspicion refers to the act of suspecting, of apprehending guilt or fault, of feeling cautiously distrustful. To distrust is to withhold trust, that is, to resist or refuse that which is desired of another. To be suspicious is thus to feel doubt, withhold, or resist feeling certain. Although suspicion is often intentional, or "directed toward objects," it is simultaneously affective because to feel suspicion is to be affected by the object with which one has contact.[3] In contrast to the word *suspicion*, the term *vaccine hesitant*, as officially used by nation-states and the medical community is defined by the WHO as the delay in acceptance or complete refusal of vaccines in the context of available immunization services.[4] In this framework, hesitancy is understood to be variously influenced by people's lack of confidence in vaccines, a perceived lack of need for or value placed on vaccines, difficulty accessing vaccines, or (dis)trust in vaccines or one's provider. Suspicion might thus be seen as the affective, more ambiguous expression of Afro-Barbadians' feelings toward the HPV vaccine, which encapsulates but transcends hesitancy in the biomedical sense. Suspicion opens Afro-Barbadians to the affective, gut feelings, and historically constituted and transnational circuits that often result in subsequent attempts to protect their children through the refusal of the HPV vaccine.

Suspicion, I am proposing, is that quality transmitted or passed on over time through the flesh and the gut, that contagious feeling complexly bound up in residual memories of the past that thrive in the present. In this sense, rather than discounting suspicion as a mere personal resistance and response to vaccination, we might understand it as that which circulates and sticks in affective economies that surround a multiplicity of socioeconomic and political formations, and also contemporary and historical biopolitical technologies, policies, and state interventions.

But what makes suspicion "stick"? How does suspicion travel in Barbados? What is its relationship to the "here and there" and the "then and now"—to the political economy and the violence of coloniality and the life-saving promises of biomedicine and citizen relationships in Barbados?[5] What encounters, commitments, and epistemologies do contagious affects invite—implore—for scholars interested in conceptualizing citizens' entangled engagements with biotechnologies like the HPV vaccine? To answer these questions, and more capaciously appreciate the fluidity with which suspicion appears to move cross-temporally in Barbados and in excess of the political economy, we need better understandings of the uneven and contradictory multiscalar economies and circuits, (post)colonial, imperial, racialized, and nationalist histories that exist in the Caribbean region, which these suspicious affects and capacities to feel encounter, surround, and travel between.

Understanding the suspicion that surrounds the HPV vaccine in Barbados involves moving spatially and temporally to capture the historical arrangements that prefigure the contemporary fiscal economies that extend across the Barbadian state to circulate around the technology of the vaccine and similar biopolitical technologies. By mapping these interconnected and transnational economies, including (but not limited to) neoliberal drives toward privatization, the Caribbean's regional economic integration into a single market and economy, an ongoing recession, and increased Barbadian government surveillance and securitization, we can better understand the ways suspicion functions outside of or in addition to a response to vaccination. That is, we can appreciate how suspicion realigns communities and refashions subjectivities in Barbados today, producing ethical encounters that occur between everyday citizens, the government of Barbados, and its representatives and that implore some citizens to protect themselves while questioning the government's accountability and true motives.

This chapter sets the framing approach for suspicion as an affective form that is implicitly bound up in the country's sociohistorical and economic fabric. It traces suspicion as it circulates in the Barbadian state and offers a broader exploration of the socioeconomic environment into which the HPV vaccine was introduced in Barbados, including the country's facilitation of intraregional migration and related government policies and engagements intended to promote economic growth and securitization. It underscores the intensity with which suspicion is distributed spatially and suffused across the Barbadian state's seemingly banal political and economic maneuvers and policies, not least of which is its public health HPV vaccination program. As suspicion differentially positions and assigns value to neoliberal technologies and products from biometric scanners to the HPV vaccine, this chapter argues, the affective engagements of citizens with these technologies are similarly affected.

Beginning with a discussion of the culture of neoliberal globalization in Barbados through the country's membership in the Caribbean Single Market and Economy, I trace the actualization of suspicion as it moves toward neoliberal arrangements such as this. Detailing nurses' and Afro-Barbadian parents' articulations of suspicion around the HPV vaccine—as just one of many government-led policies—I proceed to highlight how suspicion attaches to this biomedical technology in ways that are enmeshed in the economy, but productive of affective relations and divides that transcend the economic realm.

The Caribbean Single Market and Economy

The 1980s marked a well-established turning point in the English-speaking Caribbean away from inward-oriented and state-led development adopted in the 1960s and 1970s and toward International Monetary Fund and World Bank structural adjustment programs, the retreat of the state from nation-building, and the privileging of the free market. These developmental changes ensued in conjunction with broader crises in the world economy and the introduction of trade policies which more closely aligned with the neoliberal tenet of free market and trade liberalization. As trade liberalization increased and world markets opened, the anglophone Caribbean was forced to forgo its preferential trading agreements, trade diversions, and economic partnership agreements with European and North American markets. By the late 1980s, the entry of new competitors alongside stagnant intraregional trade resulted in dramatic declines in the manufacturing sectors of much of the Caribbean.[6] In Barbados specifically, while sugarcane cultivation previously sustained the economy, a global decline in sugarcane prices coupled with progressive liberalization and weak intra- and extraregional trade links in the 1980s left the country unable to compete in the global economy on this front. In 1989, Caribbean Community and Common Market (CARICOM) member states agreed to more comprehensive integration to expand the movement of skilled labor, capital, and services and to increase their competitiveness in the world market under the nexus of the Caribbean Single Market Economy (CSME).[7]

Like the European Union after which it was modeled, the CSME (formally launched in 2006), was a region-wide effort on behalf of eleven countries to move toward open regionalism and enhance the bargaining position of CARICOM countries amid increasingly persistent economic uncertainty and neoliberal globalization.[8] By integrating into the CSME, Barbados marked an official departure from its postindependence reliance on the nationalization of manufacturing industries and a shift toward a competitive free-market space.[9] Beyond enabling economic expansion and competitiveness by harmonizing trade laws in common market areas, the CSME accelerated the flow of production, services, and human capital. As a result, one of the major provisions was the free movement of skilled regional laborers among member states. Facilitating these flows amid complex policy regulations, competing domestic politics, and institutional capacities, however, has proved immensely difficult.

Barbados in particular faced significant challenges implementing the CSME. Shortly after becoming a signatory, its economy plunged into a deep recession on the heels of the 2008 world financial crisis, which was responsible for slowing the inflows of foreign exchange, reducing the island-recorded economic growth from 0.4 percent in 2008 to 0.2 percent in 2015, and increasing the public debt-to-gross domestic product ratio from 56 percent in 2008 to 101 percent in 2015.[10] While in 2001 the United Nations ranked Barbados's Human Development Index as 31 out of 174 countries, by 2018 it ranked the island 58th worldwide and 3rd in the Caribbean; a dramatic 27-place fall in ranking over nearly two decades.[11] Although falling international oil prices, a rebound in tourist arrivals after late 2015, and a series of austerity measures under the newly instated government in 2018 did begin to improve the country's external economic position, throughout my research trips in Barbados between 2015 and early 2018, many Barbadians claimed that sociopolitical instability and unease remained, due in part to an increase in violent crimes, societal concerns over job security, distrust in government accountability, and suspicion of intraregional migrants.

More than a decade after the official launch of the CSME, regional economic integration and full implementation into a single market and economy have failed to evolve as envisioned. Although some have touted the CSME as one of the region's only viable attempts at facilitating survival in these precarious times, some suggest we ought to examine how such regional arrangements—regardless of their successes in adapting to new neoliberal economic assemblages—are involved in manifesting neoliberal configurations and mobilities of their own.[12] This chapter illustrates how citizens' experiences of suspicion that materialize alongside configurations such as the CSME ought to be understood as circulating in the same economies as those surrounding similar state-led neoliberal policies and technologies and other proposed government technologies such as fingerprinting machines at Barbados's ports of entry.

While drives toward privatization, economic insecurity, and government indifference have had grave effects on local communities throughout the Caribbean, globalization has similarly engendered and often demanded new modes of entrepreneurship, relationality, and cultural production across the region. Pointing to the lucrative ways citizens are entering global markets and creatively forging new identities, relationships, and communities amid and often because of increasing economic uncertainty, Caribbean theorists have foregrounded the particularities of economic and social neoliberalism in an effort to challenge the dominant narrative of its deleterious effects.[13] Carla Freeman's ethnographic study on increasing modes of entrepreneurship in Barbados illustrates how the flexibility of contemporary neoliberalism has spurred the innovative move toward entrepreneurship for many middle-class citizens in the face of widespread economic precarity.[14] For Freeman, this new and pervasive entrepreneurship is not simply a mechanism of employment in the wake of widespread neoliberal policy frameworks but a form of self-making imbued with emotional expression and feeling which she argues is present across multiple spheres in the Barbadian context. Freeman characterizes these embodied feelings and emotions as affects, actively involved in the production of a new and ingenious entrepreneurial culture in Barbados, and encourages us to acquaint ourselves with these affective circuits as interpretative frames with which to approach shifting neoliberal regimes and ways of life in Barbados today. Taking this call to study affect seriously in the current context of neoliberal globalization, we might consider how suspicion circulates as affect for many Afro-Barbadians alongside arrangements and technologies as seemingly disparate as the CSME and the HPV vaccine.

Marking the thirtieth anniversary of CARICOM, the former prime minister of Barbados, Owen Arthur, noted: "The creation of a Caribbean Single Market Economy will unquestionably be the most complex, the most ambitious and the most difficult enterprise ever contemplated in our region."[15] One of the key challenges Caribbean people must overcome to successfully implement the CSME, he argues, "is the psyche . . . and the fear associated with nationals of other CARICOM countries being afforded the same rights and privileges as nationals from 'MY' country."[16] Though CARICOM laborers are legally entitled to explore cross-border opportunities in Barbados under the CSME, cross-border politics characterized by fear and attempts to securitize migration and restrict the free movement of CARICOM nationals have resulted in hostility toward intraregional migrants. Indeed, many with whom I spoke shared the popular belief that the influx of legal and illegal intraregional nationals (specifically Guyanese migrants) who came to live and work in Barbados after the official implementation of the CSME in 2006 were suspected to have exacerbated the economic recession the country has faced since 2008. Although some commentators have claimed that migrant Guyanese, Vincentian, and St. Lucian workers have in fact helped strengthen the Barbadian economy by performing the many agricultural, domestic, and construction jobs that are widely deemed undesirable by Barbadians, popular sentiment suggests otherwise.[17] My interactions with Guyanese and Jamaican migrants in Barbados further reveals an acute awareness of this purported negativity. While visiting a local market one Saturday morning, for example, a Guyanese vendor was advertising a fundraising event to support the rental of a new apartment for her and her son after their home burned down. When I inquired about how their house caught fire, she dismally proclaimed that it was likely arson because "we are Guyanese, and, they don't like us here in Barbados."

Interestingly, amid these expressions of perceived hostility toward CARICOM migrants, some have argued that Barbados has been less prohibitive toward North American and European immigrants, suggesting and reinforcing the claims of a specifically anti-CARICOM (rather than broader antiforeigner) sentiment.[18] In their report on the CSME to the Caribbean Policy Development Centre, Peter Wickham and colleagues describe CARICOM nationals' experiences traveling in the Caribbean as increasingly difficult and potentially invasive, noting, "Immigration presents the greatest hassle and the officers are overly suspicious of the region's people wanting to work illegally in other territories. Customs in Barbados was singled out as presenting significantly greater hassle to the traveler."[19] The authors are clear to differentiate between "hassle-free travel" and the "freedom of movement" that CSME promises, noting that "one can experience hassle free travel depending on the attitude of the immigration authorities, despite the fact that there are regulations with which the traveler must comply," and conversely that "one may have freedom of movement, but still experience hassles."[20]

The 2011 case of Jamaican national Shanique Myrie is testament to these claims of immigration hassles for CARICOM citizens in Barbados. On March 14, 2011, then twenty-two-year-old Myrie arrived at the Grantley Adams International Airport in Barbados, where she was denied entry and subjected to a dehumanizing and unlawful body cavity search and insults based on her Jamaican nationality. Although a search of her luggage revealed no contraband items, Myrie was detained overnight and deported to Jamaica the following day. Myrie filed a lawsuit against state of Barbados for special and punitive damages, accusing it of violating her fundamental human rights as well as rights to free movement within the Caribbean community. Though the Caribbean Court of Justice dismissed claims that Myrie suffered discrimination on the sole basis of her nationality, it awarded her US$38,620 in damages and held that CARICOM nationals "are entitled to enter CARICOM Member States, without harassment or the imposition of impediment, and stay for up to six months."[21] This public case and the many "hassles" which many CARICOM nationals (including myself) face when entering Barbados as visitors might be understood as indicative of the wider suspicions toward intraregional nationals living and working in Barbados.

Barbados Underground, a local online blog that covers controversial Barbadian news, is one of the many fora through which Barbadians frequently voice their concerns and suspicions about the CSME, intraregional migration, and

CARICOM countries' interests in Barbadian companies. In a 2012 post titled "The Hegemony of Trinidad Continues," one blogger describes the US$45 million acquisition of Barbados's Butterfield Bank by the Trinidadian-owned First Citizens Bank and claims that anti–Trinidad and Tobago sentiment is brewing in Barbados as a result of the increased influx of investors descending on the country's shores. Responses to the article highlight a distrust of CARICOM countries investing in Barbados and a sense of frustration over the passivity some Bajans claim to be witnessing among fellow citizens in light of these increasing intraregional acquisitions and rearrangements. As one reader comments, "Trinidadians own Barbados National Bank, whose name will soon be changed. . . . [They have] merged it with Barbados Mortgage Finance, which resulted in the loss of jobs for Barbadians. They have boasted about their profits, yet we complain about who sold the bank, instead of sending a message to them by withdrawing our money and put it in the credit unions, we continue to do business with them."[22] Echoing these sentiments and further condemning these new business arrangements as unfavorable though anticipated outcomes from the CSME, another commentator vents: "So what did we expect from CSME? . . . Handouts? CSME is nothing but a 21st century Trojan horse. . . . Now we have welcomed the enemy into our gates and handed them control of our news, our banks, our companies. . . . The only thing left to hand over now are our asses . . . uhhh ASSETS."[23] Beyond the sarcastic tone, such comments inadvertently allude to the suspicion I have been tracing, while notably underscoring its affective nature—that is, its potential as some capacity to act. They point to how suspicion corrals a sense of belonging through its caution against accepting the status quo and highlight how it forges ethical calls for citizens to act on the apparent threats it makes clear. Much in the same way a sense of suspicion and nonbelonging attached to me as a Trinidadian researcher, so it attached to other CARICOM nationals working and residing in Barbados, increased foreign investments in the country and other facets of the political economy—linking in particular ways to biopolitical and economic policies, practices, and technologies introduced by the government. Public skepticism around securitization attempts at ports of entry provides another useful example of suspicion's circulation and its affective nature.

Securitization and Suspicion

In 2009, the government of Barbados implemented a biometric screening program in an attempt to alleviate the threat of undocumented CARICOM nationals, criminals, and other illegal immigrants. By installing fingerprint readers at various ports of entry, the government hoped to strengthen its border security by capturing and storing the biodata of all those entering Barbados.[24] This pilot scheme was quickly abandoned due to a lack of legislation required to authorize the storage of biodata and intense local and regional resistance to this initiative variously described as undemocratic, sudden, and invasive.[25] While I visited Barbados in 2016, talk of this biometric screening program resurfaced via radio and TV announcements alerting the public that the government would be instituting mandatory fingerprinting for all persons entering and exiting Barbados as of 1 April 2016. Upon further investigation, it seemed that this biometric scheme was once again being attempted further to the 2015 Immigration (Biometrics) Regulations formulated by Prime Minister Freundel J. Stuart in his capacity as Minister Responsible for Immigration. As pursuant to Section 31 (g) and (h) of the Immigration Act, the collection of biometric data, including "facial images, fingerprints, voice or facial recognition," was thought to be particularly useful for identifying persons suspected of residing in Barbados contrary to the Immigration Act. According to Stuart, at a time when national identification cards were being falsified and criminal activity was on the rise, fingerprinting at all of Barbados's ports of entry was a necessary measure to protect citizens and their identities and the Barbados passport, which he claimed, ranked number one in the English-speaking Caribbean.[26] As before, the proposed fingerprinting scheme received intense criticism from the government's opposition party and from the Barbadian public in written commentaries and online blog contributions. As a national and regional security measure, the most recent proposal was also of concern to the wider CARICOM community, which argued it should have received prior meaningful discussion and consultation, especially with regard to the CSME and the free movement of its nationals.

In response to these criticisms, the government boasted support for this policy from the US Department of Homeland Security; for many, this further intensified their suspicions toward their government and its strategic geopolitical interests and alliances. As one citizen noted in response to an article on the proposed scheme in the *Nation News* newspaper,

> The [prime minister] seems clueless to reality. I lived in the USA, one of the most threaten[ed] countries in the world by terrorists. I travel often outside the USA [and] have never been fingerprinted or [seen] mandatory biometrics leaving or entering; the only persons [to] go through the process are visitors or resident card holders, so I believe the people should protest in the *strongest way* against citizens of Barbados going through any process of fingerprinting or mandatory biometrics. . . . [The prime minister] should

use the money more wisely to stop all the guns/drugs getting into the country killing so many people, also [to] create jobs for some of the many unemployed people. Observing this PM for a number of years now he seems to think he is [not] accountable to the people of Barbados, he can do whatever and the people have to accept; that's not a Democracy, last time I check[ed] Barbados was a Democracy [that has] a PM who is a *Public Servant * Employed by the People of Barbados. * People of Barbados "If you don't Stand for Something you'll Fall for Anything" and as Bob Marley said, "Stand Up, Stand Up, Stand Up for Your Rights."[27]

In local newspapers, others speculated that this was yet again the government mindlessly adhering to some international (most likely US) dictates and securitization measures without considering the freedoms and rights of their own citizens by implementing such an undemocratic scheme. Others expressed their suspicion over the cost and safety of this initiative. Who would citizens' biometric data be shared with should fingerprinting become mandatory? How much money would this scheme cost taxpayers? How secure would these databases be? Could personal information be hacked and used for nefarious purposes? After three months of intense public debate and legal challenges, the Immigration Department decided to defer the initiative yet again and revisit its procedures to correct irregularities.

I discuss this effort at securitization and the resistance that circulated around it because the government's impetus to implement this biometric scheme and the public response to it are wrapped in a sense of suspicion and distrust but also a desire to protect citizens' rights and opportunities. Like the HPV vaccine, information and securitization technologies such as biometric screening machines are tied to suspicion and modes of skepticism that differently affect citizens and the relations between them. It is no surprise, then, that many Barbadians whom I met spoke similarly of the HPV vaccine, the CSME and CARICOM migration, and the proposed biometric screening machines, tying these policies and technologies to violations of privacy and protection, and untrustworthy political and economic governmental maneuvers. Indeed, several of the Afro-Barbadian parents I interviewed punctuated their concerns about the HPV vaccine with criticisms of their government for prioritizing foreign prescriptions and investments over the safety of Barbadians.

Randall, a successful Afro-Barbadian business owner and father of a teenage son for whom he refused the HPV vaccine, described the government of Barbados as follows:

> I think they are puppets. . . . The government of Barbados is under the same pressure as those in other smaller countries. We decided that we don't want to condone, um . . . lemme make sure I get this right, okay, we don't want to condone buggery, it is against the law. We have our issues (like everyone else), [ours is] with homosexuality, yet we are being told that if we don't amend our laws to fall in line with the world's laws then there will be sanctions. Huh? Well, if you are going to sanction me for that, who is to say that you would not threaten me with sanctions for not agreeing to vaccines? So, they must be following others. I mean why do we always follow what Americans do?

Embedded in Randall's comments are homophobic anxieties about same-sex relations echoed by many citizens and the government. These concerns about homosexuality are deeply entangled in complex historical, colonial terrains through which power and modes of belonging are produced in Barbados, and at once ironic given the popular saying among Bajans that Barbados is in fact "90 percent gay, while others claim it is 100 percent homophobic."[28] Randall's comments also reveal the precarity of Barbados, and the concerns that citizens like him have about the government's motivations and decisions to pander to international dictates in unstable economic times. These anxieties, I suggest, can also be framed alongside concerns about the range of political and economic realignments and changes in social policy the government has undertaken since the 1990s. Amid widespread economic insecurity, many wonder, Which concerns, visions, values and plights of Barbadians will be overlooked in an attempt to align with foreign directives, trends, and/or financial incentives?

Selena, an Afro-Barbadian seamstress in her mid-thirties and legal guardian of her fourteen-year-old niece, said her niece was offered the HPV vaccine in her school in 2014. Like Randall, Selena refused the vaccine for her niece primarily because of skepticism about the government's motivations for introducing it to the Barbadian market:

> NICOLE: So, you mentioned being concerned that Merck is withholding information about the vaccine. What are your thoughts about the Barbados government?

SELENA: I think the government is well aware of what it does. I think, however, what the government does is that if [the HPV vaccine] is a requirement by your country to be part of x group, or for the UN to probably rate it at different levels to say well, this country utilizes this practice so it's on a higher level than this country or whatever, then the government is going to do whatever it needs to because it is gonna want to appear to be on a higher level or a better level or more developed than other countries. So, they will do what is supposedly required even if they don't totally agree with it. But if it's going to be better for the country in the sense that it will make it look better to the world, well . . . they're going to do it!

NICOLE: So you see the government here as wanting to project a certain image of itself?

SELENA: Yes, that's exactly how I see it. I believe that under the current government I find that we've had some uprisings and some issues here with companies that want to come and build plants, create dumps, and all kind of things like that and the government is willingly signing off on these contracts without even second-guessing or thinking about what they are really doing. They are so free and easy to let a company come and build wherever they want on our island, or import garbage into our country, and build a dump because it's gonna increase their revenue without thinking about how it's going to affect the population. [They're not thinking of] how it's gonna affect the water supply which comes from the ground, and without having those things in mind and you sign off on that then you're pretty much signing up the country for anything as far as I'm concerned. I don't have a lot of faith in my government.

Selena's and Randall's comments highlight the transnational and geopolitical resonances of the HPV vaccine. As these citizens express their concerns about the government's motives, it becomes clear how neoliberal economics, neocolonialism, and claims to citizenship traffic with the suspicion that surround the vaccine and its pharmaceutical manufacturers and promoters, much like how they do with mandatory biometric screening machines and policies such as those facilitated by the CSME. Apart from bringing into focus underlying socioeconomic issues and the affects that surround these contexts, these technologies and policies are themselves sites to which affect and its historical inhabitations stick. Examining technologies like the HPV vaccine, the pharmaceutical industry, and the discourses that surround it are thus useful modes through which we can come to understand the workings and potentialities of suspicion in postcolonial Barbados.

It is noteworthy that despite the distrust many Barbadians express of CARICOM nationals, it is overwhelmingly outsiders (albeit international tourists and predominantly white foreigners) who support the Barbadian economy. As previously noted, the rise in tourist arrivals alongside a fall in oil prices in late 2015 was largely responsible for helping Barbados begin to emerge from a seven-year recession after the 2008 financial crisis. As a resource-poor country, Barbados is increasingly dependent on tourism and international business and partnerships from software to pharmaceuticals to sustain its economy. Nonetheless, as with those around the CSME, these contentious relationships are shrouded in a sense of suspicion for many Barbadians. This dual (and purportedly necessary) sense of openness and resistance to infiltration is at stake here. While the government places increasing emphasis on tourism, there lingers a simultaneous economy of suspicion among many Barbadians in light of the overwhelming sense of interest in their island and its waters, opportunities, and indeed its people. The public response to the influence of the pharmaceutical industry in Barbados is a case in point, and it is intimately connected to the suspicion that surfaces around the pharmaceutical company Merck and the HPV vaccine Gardasil.

Barbados has become known as a "bioavailable zone," in which the government and its health ministries work alongside pharmaceutical companies, clinical trial organizations, genetics-of-disease researchers, and others to offer Barbadians as a research base for a variety of diseases, including asthma, heart disease, and cancer.[29] Although many Barbadians willingly participate in these ventures, which further purport to be lucrative for the country's economic landscape, skepticism still prevails among citizens and practitioners about the motives of such research and the value it holds for Barbadians and Barbadian medical practice. In his work on US-based asthma genetic studies conducted in Barbados, Ian Whitmarsh traces the implications of some of these pharmaceutical and medical partnerships. According to Whitmarsh, several doctors and nurses whom he interviewed affirmed genetics as valuable for biomedical research, but many simultaneously expressed ambivalence about the motives of the increasing medical genetic research that Barbados was subjected to and were skeptical about the effect these studies could have beyond scientific journals and for Barbadian patients themselves.[30] Such comments, he argues, speak to how the state, the pharmaceutical industry, and academic interests are perceived to be tied together in international practices driven from market interests.

HPV vaccination delivery in Barbados is similarly (and contentiously) possible through a biopolitical assemblage that includes a network of state resources, international public health organizations, and philanthropic agencies. Among these include the Barbadian Ministry of Health, pharmaceutical company Merck, the WHO, Pan American Health Organization, and the Barbados Cancer Society. These groups have undertaken various efforts to reduce the high cost of the vaccine, build infrastructure to deliver the vaccine, and drive advocacy campaigns that make possible new promissory ideals of what it means to be protected from HPV and its associated cancers. Although the vaccine is heavily subsidized by this nexus of state, nongovernmental, and humanitarian organizations, the fact that Gardasil is the most expensive childhood vaccine to have ever been marketed makes the biocapitalistic motivations of the manufacturers difficult (perhaps impossible) to disentangle from the medical advances the vaccine promises. Here, as with Whitmarsh's ethnographic research on genomics, the excessive biocapitalist influence of the pharmaceutical industry does not go unnoticed by Barbadian health care practitioners and citizens. In my interviews with doctors, nurses, and parents about the HPV vaccine, suspicion toward the pharmaceutical industry and its financial motives was raised continually.

Nurse Alleyne, an immunization nurse at one of the island's polyclinics, has more than two decades of experience working in public health. As we sat down to begin our interview, she said to me, "It's simple, all of this resistance to the vaccine is because people are suspicious. . . . Everything was different about the rollout and, to be honest, us nurses have just been doing damage control because of it." Over the course of an hour, in a busy room of patients and nurses, Nurse Alleyne offered a generous depiction of her experiences over the previous two years interacting with apprehensive parents, sharing some of her own concerns about the program's implementation:

When the campaign began, instead of handing the vaccine to [nurses] and allowing us to treat it as any other vaccine and introduce it to the public . . . [the ministry] started off with town hall meetings and meetings with principals of the schools and so on, and these different focus groups which were run by the Ministry of Health. . . . What I think the ministry should have done was say to us public health nurses that they have a new vaccine that they would like us to introduce to John Public and leave it to us.[31] Because we handle these people on a daily basis and we know all about the quirks and everything. So, if they had allowed the public health nurses to do their job I think that would have made a big difference. We introduced hepatitis B, no problem. We introduced MMR [measles, mumps, and rubella vaccine], no problem. We have even brought forward the MMR now from three years to eighteen months because the research pointed to an increase of measles, mumps and rubella, and again it was no problem for parents to accept. But the government, the ministry, and doctors, they just took it out of our hands and sorry to say, but when doctors feel that "I am a doctor so I must be out there in the front," it just messed up the whole thing. The doctors messed it up.

Like Nurse Dobbs, who first made clear the term *suspicious* in connection to parents' responses to the vaccine, Nurse Alleyne empathizes with citizens' feelings about the introduction of the vaccine and alludes to the frustration she and many of her colleagues had over the nontraditional way the vaccine was introduced. Emphasizing the ease with which she and other nurses have historically spearheaded vaccination campaigns in Barbados, she highlights a deep familiarity with the public and a confidence in promoting community health and safety via education, assessment, and preventative measures such as vaccination. Alleyne casts doubt not only on doctors' ability to do the same but on what she believed were their egotistical motivations for acting as the face of this noteworthy public health campaign. Others, like Nurse Riley, were more explicit in expressing the sense of suspicion they felt about how the campaign was rolled out, and specifically about the significant role Merck played in providing nurses with what she described as "materials to sell the product." According to Riley:

> One of my concerns was that they were using the vaccine's [pharmaceutical] company itself to aid in the teaching for nurses, which is generally not the case to that extent. So again for me it led to suspicion because for all the other products that we introduce, they are introduced by a team from the Ministry of Health. But it seemed more like a promotional activity, you know, like a marketing activity so that was, again [a] red flag for me.

In speaking of their personal concerns, Nurse Alleyne and Nurse Dobbs allude to how suspicion attaches for nurses, too, not just to the vaccine but to the doctors who initially spearheaded its promotion and the pharmaceutical company that manufactured it. Circulating and intensifying alongside governmental decision making, pharmaceutical interests, and Barbados's everyday politics, it appears that suspicious affects hold the potential to shape people's emotional, mental, and bodily engagements with technologies like the vaccine, as well as their relationships with the government, its involvement in transnational neoliberal assemblages, and its complicity with biopolitical campaigns and technologies. In chapter 5, I speak in more depth to the ways suspicion invades the medical profession in Barbados such that doctors also alternated between expressing ambivalence about the vaccine and denigrating doubting parents.

David is a forty-nine-year-old Afro-Bajan secondary school teacher and father of two. After leaving his house one Sunday afternoon after meeting with him and his wife, Rada, I was struck by how strongly he expressed a commitment to doing what was right for his children even when his decisions went against popular beliefs. When it came to making a decision about the HPV vaccine for his twelve-year-old daughter, Daphne, fulfilling this duty meant carefully considering all the interests at stake in the promotion of the HPV vaccine in Barbados. While he continually acknowledged the potential health benefits of the vaccine (and thus the implications it held for a reduction of cervical cancer rates), he just as firmly expressed suspicion over Merck's financial motives. Unable to reconcile these seemingly competing health and economic interests, David and Rada ultimately decided against vaccinating their daughter:

DAVID: Yeah, it seems like, well, this will contribute to the national health interest and that's the … that's the concern of government. … But at US $450 for the complete vaccine, Big Pharma making a lot of money off of this thing. You know there's a theory that the world has too many people. Big Pharma is going to solve the problem. So, AIDS, and what is the last thing they had in Africa there? Oh, Ebola, comes along. Then, all of a sudden a man had a patent for Ebola. You see, when I read these things I am like, eh heh … Big Pharma! But no, no, no, buddy, we gonna be down here for a little while longer [laughs]. We don't have any religious phobias or conspiracy theories or anything like that when it comes to drugs. It's not that we never administer drugs to our children, but … Big Pharma is mekking a lot of money out of this thing!

RADA: And to me, I didn't have it [the vaccine] and I still going strong. You go and yuh do yuh Pap smears when yuh supposed to do them, pay attention to yourself. I figure if she [Daphne] does that, she'd be able to pick up signs early if anything happens.

DAVID: And you are even more educated now than your mother.

RADA: Right, true. True.

DAVID: I don't understand the need. I mean, I mean, yes, there's a high incidence of cervical cancer in the Caribbean, but does that necessitate a government forcing you to inoculate your child, vaccinate your child? Because when they come on TV they make you appear to be stupid for not taking it. How dare you?

"How dare you?" David reiterated this question throughout our interview. Like many other parents with whom I spoke, he took offense at doctors, public health nurses, schoolteachers, and any others who sought to impose the vaccine on him and his daughter, despite the suspicions he felt obliged to take seriously. David also points to the ways he felt public health advertisements and the Ministry of Health made him feel that he was stupid for refusing the vaccine, that perhaps he lacked the education and knowledge necessary to accept the health care resources being offered. David was not alone in his views or in his insistence on following the epistemologies and questions to which suspicion led him. Time and again, parents like David connected their suspicion about the vaccine to the financial motives of Big Pharma.

Randall characterizes his distrust in pharmaceutical companies alongside his larger suspicions about health care and the global proliferation of vaccines. He and I spent a great deal of time discussing the Zika virus, of which the government had confirmed its first cases in Barbados that same week. Randall was confident that the WHO or the CDC would quickly begin discussions of a vaccine to cure Zika, even though, he claimed, it had been discovered nearly seven decades ago in Uganda. Although Randall vaccinated his son with many of the recommended childhood vaccines, he described being wary of the host of new vaccines he was seeing at the time:

> I remember twenty years ago we received a few vaccines. Now today children are getting something like thirteen, fourteen vaccines. What has really happened in that short space of time? You know, it makes you wonder. Why do we suddenly need to have this level of protection? Are we to believe that this level of protection was always warranted but we never knew it because we hadn't done enough research? Like with the situation with cancer, everybody is saying well obviously cancer is now rampant. People are wondering, is it really now rampant or are we now simply able to identify how rampant it is? So that is a bit of a tug-of-war there. . . . So I liken that to this situation now [with the HPV vaccine]. Is it that we always had issues with these ailments and they were killing us and we didn't know or are we also using this umm vaccine approach to every single thing, even things we don't even need to. Are we simply creating vaccines to finance the pharmaceutical industry? It's business, you know. It's business. So I am always very skeptical about things like that because of the things I've seen these powers do. I don't put it past them for this to be another part of their plot. So all this would have been fueling my thoughts behind the [HPV] vaccine.

Although Randall's comments and many of the excerpts herein are examples of subjectively experienced shifts and emotions, they can be mapped alongside nurses' suspicions of doctors, of the vaccine's unique rollout, of citizens' concerns around biometric screening machines, and Barbadians' ambivalence toward various state efforts and biopolitical efforts. These affective economies of suspicion activate subjectivities, forms of relationality, and knowledge/ethics in contemporary Barbados. Suspicion opens citizens like Randall, David, and Rada to different types of questions, narratives, and forms of knowledge that conflict with those of the government and the pharmaceutical industry working toward HPV vaccine promotion and acceptance and disconnects them from the ideas, people, and objects they deem untrustworthy. As will be detailed in the coming chapters, affects of suspicion ought to be understood as productive—generative of multiple and multiply conceived communities and imaginings of protection and care despite and alongside their fraught repercussions.

Conclusion

In her review of Carla Freeman's book *Entrepreneurial Selves* on entrepreneurialism, affect, and neoliberalism in Barbados, Caribbean feminist and political economist Peggy Antrobus reflects on the sustainability of the tenacious entrepreneurship that Freeman argues permeates Barbados in the twenty-first century.[32] Antrobus questions its social effects at a time when the confidence of virtually all of the country's economic sectors has been shaken and the government at the time widely deemed undependable. Can an economy that is oriented toward individualism and small business truly foster a sense of community?[33] In Barbados in 2016, Antrobus and I discussed some of these issues in relation to this research around HPV and suspicion. As I have done throughout this chapter, I suggested to her that the often negatively perceived "hesitancy"—or affects of suspicion I was observing to circulate in Barbados—did in fact make up distinct economies and communities, even if they were fashioned in unintentional and (some would correctly argue) undesirable and potentially dangerous ways.

As Freeman notes, through affects (such as intimacy) that can be widely observed in Barbados today, "not only are markets and products and services being refashioned and realigned, so too are gender, class, cultural and racial subjectivities being reconstituted."[34] Although the affect of suspicion I describe in this book differs in that it also espouses disconnect and nonbelonging with suspicious objects and groups, it nonetheless embodies forms of meaning, belonging, and connection for the groups of citizens who make meaning from the ethical imperatives it engenders. Suspicion, I argue, is neither a private nor an individual feeling. Instead, by means of sticky associations over time and in space, suspicion aligns some Bajans together in ways that are disconnected from pharmaceutical companies, doctors, intraregional residents, and at times researchers and visitors like myself.

While suspicion's potential to engender parents' refusal of the HPV vaccine inevitably threatens public health attempts to save lives via vaccination, this book offers insight into the undertheorized ways that suspicion is also generative for public health practitioners and academics. It details how suspicion instills in Afro-Barbadian parents ethical imperatives and epistemologies of care and protection, not just from the vaccine and its unknown side effects but against the perceived financial motivations of government–industry partnerships and centuries-long modes of material and ideological violence under the guise of biopolitics, while holding the state accountable for the well-being of its citizens.

Although novel in their current appearance, modes of digital surveillance and administration, technologies like the HPV vaccine and biometric screening machines, and the policies through which they are brought to the Barbadian public also have deep political and sordid histories that are enmeshed in colonial biopolitics of public health, policing, and foreign extraction. Chapter 2 examines a range of these histories in which suspicion, risk, and biopolitics have circulated and continue to reside in Barbados and the anglophone Caribbean.

TWO

Risk and Suspicion: An Archive of Surveillance and Racialized Biopolitics in Barbados

In the 1980s, sociologist Ulrich Beck famously coined the term *risk society* to refer to the widespread social preoccupation with and intensive management of risk across industrial societies.[1] As a modern concept, risk refers to "calculating the incalculable, colonizing the future," in which danger and peril are associated less with demons, nature, and gods and more with "*un*natural, human-made, manufactured uncertainties and hazards."[2] The history of risk, however, precedes these contemporary understandings, originating in the financial realm of transnational maritime insurance and commercialism. In seventeenth- and eighteenth-century maritime history (and, indeed, maritime slavery), risk referred to a material and corporeal "financial instrument for coping with the mere *possibility* of peril, hazard or danger."[3] To cope with the natural "perils of the seas" or an "act of God," colonial merchants would purchase financial compensation or insurance on their risks (including human risks of the enslaved).[4]

As the concept of risk became popularized in the English language from the late eighteenth century (coinciding with rise of capitalism), so did understandings of risk as something at once material, extreme, immaterial, and in need of quantification and management. Across Europe and the United States, risk management mushroomed in the form of new financial institutions, stock markets, savings accounts, and insurance companies, the latter of which eventually began adopting statistical approaches to mathematically predict chronic disease susceptibilities of prospective policy holders.[5] During this time, risk discourse and theorization entered the arena of medicine with statistical aggregations increasingly used to scientifically and mathematically quantify uncertainty around disease transmission. By the 1830s, statistics had entered squarely into the field of public health. Drawn on for its ability to evaluate and diagnose the efficacy of medical treatment, statistics enabled doctors, hygienists, and medical administrators to transcend a long-standing reliance on individual cases to attend to those of the population deemed most at risk; to quantify, calculate, and control probabilities around diseases; and to advise on the effect of social and environmental factors and sanitation measures.[6]

By this time, risk assessment had also become prevalent in the realm of biomedicine, where it was used to evaluate the potential dangers of new medical innovations, which have always spawned their own risks, questions about efficacy, and social understandings of how these risks might be mitigated.[7] Medical historians have detailed how these multiple configurations of risk, probability, and care and competing beliefs about a progressive modernity converged across class around interventions such as the selective use of anesthesia in Europe in the 1840s, the contraceptive pill, and vaccines—disputes over which can be traced as far back as eighteenth-century debates over smallpox inoculation in England.[8] Indeed, although public health concerns around vaccination refusal have heightened through the 2000s with the resurgence of vaccine-preventable communicable diseases in North America and Europe especially, as Nik Brown incisively notes, "vaccination [was] from its very incipient opening moments . . . inherently a precarious political affair underpinning a new biopolitics of population vitality, statehood and colonialism."[9] In addition to early European concerns around smallpox variolation, skepticism over the clinical evidence for the bacille Calmette-Guérin (BCG) tuberculosis vaccine in France and Germany and related concerns around the role that BCG vaccination campaigns in the 1950s and 1960s British Caribbean played in reinvigorating the British empire exemplify the continued tenuous history of vaccination through the twentieth century.[10] Across these examples, scientists', medical professionals', or states' rights to subject individuals to the risks of vaccination are rationalized by diminishing risk at the level of the population, and the construction of social risk factors and at-risk groups is drawn on to justify what were the then-unknown risks of vaccines.[11]

Central to these logics of risk reduction is the bio-logic of biopower, described by Foucault as the power over life. Like other reproductive technologies, vaccines act simultaneously on biopower's two poles in that the anatomo-politics or the disciplining and objectifying of individual bodies is articulated alongside the biopolitical collective regulation of populations.[12] Public resistance to vaccination emphasizes both the complexity this entwined anatomo-biopolitics presents to the public and the often disconcerting affect embedded in its disciplinary regulation. Indeed, although the utilitarian and population-based public health rationale for vaccination is publicized to reduce individual risk (even if it entails greater immediate risk) and induce herd immunity (which ultimately reduces individual risk), scientific statements and biopolitical public health policies around vaccination are not neutral, "embody[ing] and at the same time, often obscur[ing] underlying moral values and implicit political decisions."[13] To be sure, as contemporary biopower manifests increasingly through imperatives toward neoliberal self-government, individual choice, freedom, and encouragement to accept biotechnologies like the HPV vaccine as a means of caring for oneself and others, there is an increasing slippage between expert scientific, state, and industry knowledge about risk and the moral regulation of health and its relationship with factors such as race, gender, sexuality, and capital.[14] In the context of Barbados, these overlapping ideologies and interests are laid bare in public health efforts to promote the HPV vaccine.

Consider this flyer (figure 2.1), which I came across in 2016, posted to Instagram by Gyn-A-Thon Barbados (then Globeathon Barbados)—a chapter of an international movement that seeks to increase global awareness of women's gynecological cancers through outreach, education, and engagement. The flyer, which has since circulated numerous times on Instagram and Facebook, aims to raise awareness about HPV, promote the HPV vaccine as a preventative tool, and publicize the movement's annual 5K walk/run fundraising event. It declares HPV to be a common disease that nearly all sexually active women and men acquire in their lifetimes and makes explicit that high-risk strains of the disease may lead to genital warts and cancers—specifically cervical cancer in which more than 90 percent of cases are attributed to HPV. The movement's logo appears in the top right corner, and in the top left, hovering behind the text, is the torso of a white woman whose hands are placed in a heart shape over her abdomen. Social media handles are listed at the base of the flyer to direct viewers to follow the movement's multiple platforms, and posted beneath the flyer as a comment on the post are the hashtags #GlobeathonBarbados and #GetYourDaughtersVaccinated.

Since its inception in 2013, country head of Gyn-A-Thon Barbados Dr. Vikash Chatrani has been an ardent champion for the fight against gynecological cancers in Barbados and is a well-known advocate for the HPV vaccine. He noted that the 2019 rebrand of Globeathon to Gyn-A-Thon was an attempt to "give honor and pride to the female reproductive organs ... [and to] talk about

WHAT IS HPV?

The Human Papilloma Virus (HPV) is so common that nearly all sexually active men and women get it at some point in their lives. There are many different types of HPV, some of which can cause health problems including genital warts and cancers. HPV infection appears to be involved in the development of more than 90% of cervical cancer cases. **BUT** there are vaccines that can stop these health problems from happening.

  @GlobeathonBarbados Globeathon Barbados

Liked by **ced_rol** and **others**

gynathonbarbados #GlobeathonBarbados
Come out! Walk with us and Support September
11th!!! #GetYourDaughtersVaccinated

FIGURE 2.1 Globeathon promotional flyer. Posted to Instagram, September 1, 2016. Screenshot by author.

them with dignity and respect, because these organs bring all humanity to life."[15] Speaking at the rebranding launch, Dr. Dorothy Cooke-Johnson, president of the Barbados Cancer Society, echoed Chatrani's claims. Further lauding the financial company Sagicor Life for its five-year sponsorship of the movement, she commented on the privilege that came with working with "the best company in Barbados," one that not only offered life/health insurance policies but was deeply invested in the health of women and dedicated to raising awareness about women's cancers.[16]

Together, this Instagram promotional flyer and these doctors' pointed comments index the deeply entwined configurations of risk with sexual and reproductive politics, race, gender, finance, and public health, all of which complexly surround HPV and the HPV vaccine in Barbados and warrant further exploration. For example, what meanings shall we attribute to the use of a white woman's body in the flyer to promote an event for a population that is more than 90 percent Black? How precisely is HPV being presented as a gendered disease, despite text to suggest its nondiscriminatory nature? Of what significance is it that the financial company Sagicor, which offers life and health insurance policies, is the official sponsor of Gyn-A-Thon Barbados's initiative to bring awareness to gynecological cancers and minimize their risk? What counts as risk(y) for these various constituents? How have risk and Black women's sexuality been profoundly entangled across time in the history of Barbados and the anglophone Caribbean, in their respective genealogies, and in relation to global health care and biopolitics?

I turn to these questions first by way of a brief discussion of the logics of risk, race, and capital that surround the HPV vaccine in Barbados. Highlighting the manifold politics of Black women's sexuality, medical imperialism, care, and protection that inhere in Afro-Barbadian parents' claims to suspicion around the HPV vaccine, I proceed to reflect on the multiple ways risk and suspicion have historically circulated around enslaved Black women and continue to mediate Black women's sexuality in relationship to the HPV vaccine in Barbados. Specifically, I trace how these logics were mobilized to legitimate the racialized biopolitical techniques and policies introduced by colonial officials through the postemancipation period to "save" Black women and eradicate the risks their reproductive or diseased bodies were perceived to pose. I focus on the emergence of contagious disease hospitals in Barbados in the 1860s, concerns over working-class women's bodies in the postwar period, and the introduction of birth control campaigns of the 1950s and 1960s in the anglophone Caribbean. Across these examples, I trace how suspicion crosses a range of biopolitical policies and inquiries enacted to manage risk and secure capital, much as it does for many Afro-Barbadian parents around HPV and its vaccine.

Risk, Race, Capital, and HPV Vaccination in Barbados

As a medical technology invested in protecting against HPV and its associated diseases, the HPV vaccine is both a profit-making and risk-managing device. At US$150 per shot, it provides a lucrative market for Merck while representing a scientific breakthrough as one of the first preventative cancer vaccines to be developed.[17] Often referred to as the cervical cancer vaccine, Gardasil is most popularly advertised as providing protection to young women against HPV and the risks of cervical cancer posed by the virus. But because HPV is a sexually transmitted disease, the vaccine further participates in an economy of biopolitical surveillance concerned with caring for and managing the risks of sex— preventing disease while constituting markets of risk and risk management and the surveillance of those to whom this risk attaches. In the context of Barbados, as articulated to me by nurses, Afro-Barbadian parents, and teenagers, these risks are seemed to attach disproportionately to Black adolescent girls' bodies and their sexuality. In turn, suspicion that surrounds the HPV vaccine and its administration in Barbados similarly converges around the entangled factors of risk, care, profit, science, and Black women's sexuality. Conjoined through colonial and postcolonial biopolitical techniques and technologies, these are factors that have long warranted suspicion in the colonial history of the Caribbean. Contextualizing Barbadian parents' suspicion toward the HPV vaccine and its administration thus requires a deeper understanding of how these fraught histories and politics of risk, care, and surveillance, as well as biotechnologies like vaccines, have come into being in co-constitutive ways that underlie the capitalist economy in which the HPV vaccine participates. Indeed, the very existence of the HPV vaccine in Barbados and elsewhere remakes the idea of risk (and what it means to be risk-free) into a form of capital, creating new markets for private companies to profit from and market themselves alongside.[18] Here we might think of not only pharmaceutical companies involved in manufacturing HPV vaccines but also companies like Sagicor, the corporate sponsor of Gyn-A-Thon's initiative to raise awareness of gynecological cancers and the HPV vaccine in Barbados. Like Gyn-A-Thon, and in an attempt to manage the risks of HPV and the characterization of these risks as intimately connected to sex, the Barbadian Ministry of Health predominantly promotes the vaccine to parents as a *cervical cancer* risk-reducing, life-saving technology. Despite its efforts to circumvent attention on female sexuality, risk attaches disproportionately to the adolescent female body.[19] By managing these risks through vaccine bio-technology and its accompanying modes of medical and pharmaceutical adver-tisements, public health and television broadcasting, town hall meetings, and parent-teacher meetings, the adolescent female body is subjected to increased forms of surveillance.

Echoing logics of reproductive and sexual management, the vaccination cam-paign, its economic entanglements, surveillance of female sexuality, and forceful promotion travel through disturbing racialized pasts in the country's history. The government's medicopharmaceutical HPV vaccination campaign, designed to manage these risks of sex, becomes shrouded in suspicion for Afro-Caribbean parents in particular, for whom risk takes on multiple meanings—attaching not just to HPV but to the vaccine and its administrators who work on behalf of the postcolonial state and in a legacy of biopolitical experimentation on Afro-Caribbean women throughout the colonial period. For many of the parents with whom I spoke, the risks to be managed around HPV lay not simply around their daughters' budding sexual activity and exposure to the virus but around the state's claims to biopolitics offered in the all-too-familiar name of care and protection. For these parents, the perceived risks with accepting the HPV vac-cine were further intensified by the climate of economic precarity and social un-ease that permeated Barbados during my research period from 2015 to 2018—a time when citizens were not only frustrated with but suspicious of their govern-ment and its strategic biopolitics amid widespread apathy, financial cutbacks, and neglect in major sectors from education to employment since the global economic crisis of 2008.

Danielle, a forty-nine-year-old Afro-Barbadian mother, was incredibly self-reflexive in describing her suspicions about the HPV vaccine. Despite her even-tual decision to accept the vaccine for her daughter, she remained ambivalent about this choice, noting her concern about the motives that underlay the gov-ernment's decision to promote the vaccine, and its entwined financial interests with pharmaceutical companies which, she noted, have notoriously experi-mented on vulnerable Black populations across history:

> Listen, I have read a lot about how vaccines have been used to do experimen-
> tation on Black people. Of course, that will and should make me suspicious.
> And at the same time, I look at someone who will refuse a measles vaccine
> and call them stupid. Do people call me stupid for questioning the HPV vac-
> cine? [*laughs*] Maybe. But listen, the measles vaccine is tried and true. The
> HPV vaccine only targets a few strains of HPV, and there are so many other
> strains that can lead to cancer. So I'm thinking well why are you only going

after these two [strains]? I am not fully convinced this will help our girls and what is most likely to affect them in Barbados, so I found out actually in reading up more recently that the Gardasil is not really targeting the same types of HPV we have a lot of here in Barbados. And I have heard about Gardasil 9 which is I think more strains, but we are not getting that.

There are so many sneaky things that the pharmaceutical companies do that it makes you afraid to trust them sometimes. . . . I am not sure that the interest of humankind is taking precedence. I am also afraid of the government's interest here. . . . If you are in a position where someone comes to you and says, "Hey, I want to bring this vaccine to your country, I will make this worth your while" . . . well, I have fears with that. And so my hackles raise because of these types of things and alliances, right. This is the reality. And you know, I understand that giving people this vaccine can help our costs in the long run, like taking off costs of health care long-term if people aren't as sick, but I mean this vaccine I know is not cheap. And at this time when the economy is suffering and the children are also suffering in different ways because of inattention to lots of areas like schools, some of us are wondering what is really going on.

Reflecting on her criticism of those who refuse the MMR vaccine, Danielle suggests a certain level of irony in her own ambivalence toward the HPV vaccine and simultaneously defends her suspicion as significant and emergent in the face of longer histories of biomedical and pharmaceutical experimentation and profit and the overwhelming sense of economic precarity in which she and many Barbadians were living. Further questioning the government's decision to introduce a vaccine that appeared ill-suited to the population, Danielle speculates that the economic profits derived from state-industry partnerships drove this vaccination campaign, rather than the health and needs of Barbadians. Here she is referencing the use of the quadrivalent Gardasil vaccine, which covers HPV strains 6, 11, 16, and 18, with the latter known to cause approximately 70 percent of all cervical cancer cases. As Danielle correctly notes, there are important differences between the most prevalent high-risk strains of HPV in the Caribbean and those in North America and Europe. For instance, across populations of Barbadian, Trinidadian, and Jamaican women, the African-Caribbean Cancer Consortium reports that HPV 45 (rather than HPV 16 or 18) is the most commonly high-risk cervical HPV type detected.[20] In Barbados specifically, research has indicated a prevalence of HPV 45, followed by HPV 16, 52, 58, 66, and 35.[21] Though the quadrivalent vaccine (which was being offered through the national vaccination program during my time in Barbados) does offer some degree of cross-protection against other strains of HPV, these data support the value of a more accelerated introduction of Gardasil 9 in places like Barbados and other Caribbean countries. This vaccine creates more than 90 percent protection against cervical cancer associated with nine of the most common HPV types (6, 11, 16, 18, 31, 33, 45, 52, 58). Across her discussion of the country's economic precarity, the financial profits and motives of the state and pharmaceutical industries in the promoting the vaccine, and her suspicions vis-à-vis the history of medical experimentation on Black people, Danielle underscores the entwined logics of risk, race, and capital that surround the HPV vaccine and her suspicions of this biotechnology, despite her eventual acceptance of the vaccine for her daughter.

I interviewed Natty in April 2018, one month before the Barbadian elections, which resulted in the landslide victory for the Barbados Labour Party and the election of Mia Mottley, the country's first female prime minister. A thirty-four-year-old Afro-Barbadian mother of three, Natty declined the HPV vaccine for her eligible teenage son and preteen daughter. Like Danielle, she expressed suspicions about her government's priorities amid a turbulent economy and further emphasized how economic, racial, and class inequalities factor into her feelings and decision-making process about the vaccine:

> The government does not do enough. . . . Whether Party A or Party B is in power, I still gotta get up in the morning and look after me and mine, right? . . . I would like to see the lower and middle classes being able to afford housing, the basic things. As much as I think I struggle sometimes, I am well aware there are people out there doing way worse than I am, who are really wanting for food and shelter in this country. [The government] needs to make things more accessible for the lower and middle classes, right? Make it more feasible for people like me, a single mother to apply for loans for homes. . . . And so I'm not going to lie to you, I do sometimes think about what the reason is for bringing this vaccine here to Barbados. I don't want to believe that the government or any pharmaceutical company is manufacturing something that has the potential to harm people, but, like, money speaks. Is there some interest in killing out the lower-class, Black population? Who are those accepting this? I'm not going to lie; I do have thoughts like this sometimes though I keep them to myself. You see, if it was that the government said that [the vaccine] was mandatory then I would suppose that this is ultimately what is the best thing for all Barbadians, right? But when they tell us we could opt in or opt out then I am right away a little skeptical and thinking maybe it is not tested fully. The government ought to make sure it is safe, especially for our girls. That is the root of everything—motherhood—we have

to make sure that our daughters' reproductive systems are in order to bring life. Obviously, I wouldn't want it to jeopardize any other part of my daughter, but especially this. You know what I mean?

Drawing on her lived experiences of governmental neglect as a self-described struggling, middle-class Afro-Barbadian single mother, Natty questions the Barbadian state's motives in promoting Gardasil in light of its many shortcomings and inabilities to provide for the most vulnerable. Wary about the vaccine's voluntary status in light of public health messaging around the product as safe, beneficial, and necessary, she confesses to privately speculating that Barbadians who occupy similar racial and economic categories are particularly susceptible to abuse by pharmaceutical companies seeking to test their drugs. Like many of the other parents and nurses whom I interviewed, Natty questions which categories of Barbadians were readily accepting the vaccine, gesturing to how both racial and class dynamics are reflected in many parents' understandings of the risks around HPV and subsequent reception of the vaccine.

Her suspicions connect with claims by practitioners like Nurse Dobbs, who stressed that Barbados was a "close-knit" society wherein (predominately white) upper-middle-class parents held a lot of influence on others who were unsure about the vaccine: "What you basically saw was that [some lower-class parents would think] . . . I am watching you, I am looking up to you and if you are not going to give it to your child then I am not going to give it to mine. 'Why the "upper class" not giving it to theirs?' they are wondering. So if those persons are refusing, [then] there is no way they are giving it to their child. Yep, that's the Barbadian culture." Echoing Dr. Chatrani's claims regarding Gyn-A-Thon and the importance and pride we must attribute to women's reproductive organs that "bring life to all humanity," Natty is also acutely concerned with potential side effects of the vaccine on young Black girls and their ability to reproduce more generations. Not only does heteronormativity loom large here in the expectations of women's sexuality via the family and children as the future of humanity, but these comments amplify how the risks of HPV disproportionately attach to women's sexuality. As in the flyer posted to Instagram (figure 2.1), I noted that parents and health care practitioners alike focus their concerns and attention on female reproduction and cervical cancer, despite HPV's transmission across sex. While the body of a white woman is curiously used in this Gyn-A-Thon flyer to call attention to cervical cancer and female reproduction and promote the HPV vaccine, Afro-Barbadian parents like Danielle and Natty accentuate that it is Blackness and Black women's bodies like those of their daughters for whom risk and the pharmaceutical technology of the HPV vaccine hold special significance. Indeed, in articulating their suspicions, they trace the connections between race and risk as they relate to the HPV vaccine and histories of biopolitical and pharmaceutical neglect and between the Barbadian government's promotion of the vaccine, its industry alliances, and potential related economic motives. Such suspicions ought to be contextualized in the capitalist, racialized, and biopolitical history of transatlantic slavery and colonialism (which I turn to next) to underscore the logics of risk, the imperative to study Black women as risk(y), and the role of biopolitics/biomedicine in mitigating these risks over time in Barbados and the anglophone Caribbean.

Risk, Hesitancy, and Biopolitical Care in Colonial Barbados

As sociologist Mimi Sheller argues, to comprehensively analyze practices of citizenship, self-determination, and politics in the postemancipation Caribbean, one must trace the "political 'mechanisms of life': sex, pregnancy, births, longevity, health," all of which were central to the colonial project.[22] As the predominant tools of classification and spatial governance in the colonial period and into the postemancipation period in the British Caribbean, biopolitical initiatives and medicoscientific conceptualizations of racial difference were strategically employed to monitor enslaved peoples' (and especially enslaved women's) health risks so as to maximize their speculative value as laborers and human commodities.[23]

In places like Barbados, "scientifically" racist ideologies of Black people as a socially inferior, immoral species were simultaneously drawn on by merchant-planters and other white elites as a rationale for withholding and conserving the state's economic, welfare, and biopolitical resources for those deemed worthier of care.[24] Subsequently, whether it was short-lived infant pronatalist campaigns designed to foster optimal conditions for the reproduction of a Black labor supply, contagious disease hospitals deemed necessary to regulate promiscuous Black women, attempts to examine and study their reproductive labor and heterosexual comportment in the post–World War II period, or birth control campaigns aimed at encouraging their sexual control as a mark of self-governance and civility, biopolitical campaigns in Barbados and across the wider anglophone Caribbean have historically remained entangled with and predicated on the ambivalent relationship between the surveillance and care of Black women, their risky bodies, and actions.[25] Such campaigns were executed and managed with technologies of surveillance, which were at once biopolitical and necropolitical—focused on caring for, optimizing, and controlling the risks of/posed to Black women's lives through coercive and often violent, life-threatening measures, for the purposes of labor. The sustained economic calculus, capitalistic motivations, and rationales for care that undergird these differentially constituted risks and the resulting biopolitical moves enacted in response are noteworthy markers of the historically ambivalent manifestation of care and its enmeshment in the bio-logic of slavery's sordid systems.

The history of the colonial management of reproduction and childbearing reveals the pertinent risks Black women's sexuality in particular posed to colonizers during the colonial period—a risk that was simultaneously physical (through the feared spread of venereal diseases) and psychic (through its supposed ability to morally taint the British empire). As the 1807 abolition of the slave trade loomed near, the reproductive capabilities of enslaved women were acute sources of anxiety and promise for plantation overseers across the British Caribbean.[26] Through this biopolitical scheme, enslaved women were incentivized to reproduce with the promise of reformed working conditions and small monetary contributions if they successfully delivered and cared for children up to one month of age.[27] As Katherine Paugh highlights, however, though "abolitionists and plantation owners alike had frequently touted their benevolence and concern toward child-bearing women on West Indian plantations during the late eighteenth and early nineteenth centuries ... [i]n its execution, the drive to remold the reproduction of the plantation labor force was much more punitive than compassionate."[28] Although these seemingly benevolent gestures of care protected pregnant women from excessive physical labor and improved their levels of postnatal care, they simultaneously resulted in the heightened surveillance and exploitation of Black women's bodies and reproductive lives.[29] This intensified surveillance coincided with the rise of biomedicine and public health in the British empire at the turn of the century, both of which became predominant (albeit strategically deployed) colonial tools of governance after abolition and into the postemancipation period.[30]

Although it was widely agreed that infant mortality posed a threat to the economic survival of the anglophone Caribbean region after emancipation, Victorian racial attitudes and eugenicist beliefs greatly influenced theories about the causes of child mortality and often the way it should be addressed. In the eyes of many members of the white Barbadian community, it was considered neither abnormal nor inappropriate for Afro-Barbadian infants to die of malnutrition and disease due to their perceived-to-be-unfit, sexually voracious parents, who were thought to lack the innate ability to be moral and responsible.[31] Beginning in 1834, the government of Barbados introduced a series of punitive poor laws and subsidiary bastardy clauses that formalized such thinking, establishing lower-class Barbadians as physically and morally responsible for their children and criminalizing "the desertion of bastards" through emigration or other means.[32] Poor Black mothers, in particular, were held accountable through such racialized laws for the costs of their sexual irresponsibility outside the confines of marriage, and their children were viewed as resulting risks and costs to the colonial state. Managing these risks was less about addressing the decrepit social and health conditions that plagued the Black working class than it was about criminalizing those to whom risk attached through the surveillance and criminalization of Black families and infant mortality.[33]

Through the 1800s, colonial doctors, planters, and members of the legislative government in the British Caribbean continued to view poor sanitation, poverty, and widespread cholera epidemics as indistinguishable from the suspicious morals and lewd sexual behavior of Black women, who were similarly blamed for the spread of venereal diseases. Not only was physical infection thought to emanate from Black people's bodies; officials feared that their multiple risks of disease, promiscuity, and hypersexuality would afflict and morally taint the British.[34] Responsive colonial strategies to regulate and control the risks of Black and colonized people through the logics of "science," social science, and biomedicine were persistently gendered efforts to produce and instill morality and civility under the guise of biopolitical care and salvation.[35] For instance, under the supposed goal of managing the risks of syphilis, the Barbadian colonial regime sought to control Afro-Barbadian women's sexuality and discipline their bodies through the conjoined employment of law, force, and biomedicine. After mounting concerns about the risks posed to the labor supply and the health of British sailors from infected Black women, Contagious Diseases Acts (CDAs) were passed in Barbados in 1868.[36] As legislation designed to protect white male bodies from the risks of Afro-Caribbean sex workers, CDA laws stipulated that police officers could enforce power over any woman suspected of being a sex worker by issuing a certificate mandating that she receive a medical examination by British doctors to clear her of infection with venereal disease.[37] Established in 1860, the Bridgetown Contagious Disease Hospital (CDH) became the official home to which suspicious women who were believed to hold the greatest threats to the health of the British would be remanded. Such hospitals were central to enforcing the moral and regulatory work of the CDAs. As Denise Challenger notes, physicians played a key role in transforming Black women from patients to prisoners in the Barbadian hospital, wherein the risks of venereal disease discursively and disproportionately attached to young Black women of the lowest socioeconomic class: "The doctor—by virtue of his race, gender and class—had the power, if he so desired, to control the women through the pain he exerted as he prodded their sexual parts for signs of [venereal diseases]. . . . In order to function as an effective imperial and colonial tool for sexual regulation, the CDH was slowly transformed from a place of 'benign' healing into one of coercive discipline."[38] As a means of punishment and control, the very existence of the CDH ensured that even women who were not participating in sex work regulated their sexual behavior so as to assuage any suspicions that might attach to them. Along with the CDAs, the Barbadian CDH enforced and established contentious relationships between the state, Black women, and their sexuality, which continued into the twentieth century, long after the CDH was shut down in 1887.[39] Though these are only two examples of the sustained economic calculus, capitalistic motivations, and rationales for care that undergird these supposed risks of Blackness across nineteenth-century Barbados highlight the uniform convergence of suspicion and biopolitical surveillance around Black women, sexuality, and reproduction. Through the 1900s and into the postwar period in the anglophone Caribbean, suspicion continued to attach to the Black body in shifting but persistently gendered and classed ways and the management of these risks revolved increasingly around the surveillance, social, and scientific study of Black women, sexuality, and motherhood. The Moyne Report offers another illustrative case.

In 1938, in response to mounting civil unrest in the British Caribbean over state apathy, precarious economies, widespread unemployment, and the rampant spread of communicable diseases, the Crown appointed a series of citizens under the West India Royal Commission (Moyne Commission) to travel to the colonies and ascertain the social and political causes of social uprisings, hear testimony, and develop a comprehensive report on the colonies' main problems and needs.[40] So damning were the findings that the report's publication was withheld for six years until after World War II had ended in 1945, for fear that evidence of imperial negligence would lead to international criticism, dampened support for the war, or further uprisings.[41] In Barbados, the commissioners' findings confirmed the rampancy of tropical diseases, malnutrition, and overcrowding, all of which it linked to illegitimacy, the "disorganized" Black family, single mothers, and female poverty in particular. The commission feared that the then high birth rate in Afro-Caribbean communities, coupled with a declining death rate, would result in further problems for the island's population density and precarious economy. Such racist interpretations about the causes of overpopulation and commissioners' suggestions to arrange campaigns against "the social, moral and economic evils of promiscuity" echoed racist theories of disease causation held by colonial and local physicians for over a century.[42] Rather than a doomed eugenic inheritance, however, commissioners argued that socialization was to blame for the ills of the lower-class Black family and the risks they posed to the advancement of the colonies.

In line with long-standing efforts at reproductive management of Black women's sexuality, attributing overpopulation to Black laborers soon enough became the means "by which colonial officials proposed tactics such as mass sterilization of Afro-Caribbean people and the promotion of birth control to prevent overpopulation of people who were purportedly incapable of the rational restraint required to curb their sexual and reproductive impulses."[43] Following the commission's inquiry, the risks and problems of the lower-class Black family and patterns of Caribbean kinship squarely entered the academic research agenda and debate in the Caribbean from the 1950s.[44] During this period, suspicions about Black women's sexuality, motherhood, heterosexual comportment, and reproductive labor were again refixed as objects of risk to be managed via study and surveillance for the threats they posed to population growth, increasingly precarious Victorian values of respectability, strong family homes, and gender roles alike.

In the aftermath of the Moyne Report and in this postwar, preindependence context of social unrest and colonial anxiety, birth control campaigns emerged in the anglophone Caribbean. Anxieties around dangerous working-class fertility and its effect on socioeconomic and political stability were particularly acute for white elites in Barbados and Jamaica during this period, and its management through birth control was deemed a simple and necessary remedy.[45] The overwhelming support for birth control appeared to mark a sudden shift in colonial interest in the biopolitical governance of the Black working class throughout the Caribbean.[46] Black fertility and facilitating the reproduction of enslaved people had always been critical elements of colonial calculus, but never before had family practice and the control of sexuality been such a deliberate focus of the Barbadian white elites' biopolitical attention and intervention—even when it was in the name of the island's social and economic stability. Still, in these new campaigns, the explicit language of scientific and eugenic racism used to denigrate Black men and women for the past hundred years as "unfit" and "feebleminded" coalesced with pathologizing discourses in which the Black family was a threat to be controlled, studied, and managed via birth control. In places like Jamaica, this surveillance of working-class women's sexuality also took the form of research studies by US social scientists interested in studying the reproductive desires, beliefs, and behaviors of working-class women, with the aim of reducing their perceived suspicion of and resistance toward family planning.[47] Linking their support of these studies and the promotion of birth control to progressive nationalist and socialist ideals and projects, Black middle-class politicians, professionals, and reformist elites further hoped to encourage and persuade working-class women to choose birth control in the name of self-respect, nation-building, and self-governance. In this way, as Bourbonnais notes, "birth control became tied from early on to a wide variety of—at times converging, at times conflicting—agendas."[48]

In 1955, Barbados was the first country in the anglophone Caribbean (and in the entire Western Hemisphere) to establish a nationally sanctioned and supported family-planning program under the Barbados Family Planning Association (BFPA).[49] The BFPA quickly rose to become a forerunner in establishing family planning programs that were both voluntary and government run.[50] Its story is widely recognized to be one of the most successful models of government-supported family planning—one that did not coerce but encouraged the use of birth control through persuasive political discourse. Despite the steady reduction of birth rates in Barbados from the mid-1950s, long-standing colonial medicoracialized constructions and suspicions of Black women as hyperfecund and hypersexual continued to circulate through the 1960s, promulgating the fixation on working-class Black women's sexuality as a risk and threat to nation-building.[51]

Indeed, through birth control campaigns, Black middle-class leaders in Barbados were able to successfully forge social and political consensus on the necessity of contraception for the health and wealth of the country while maintaining a critique of the inequality and domination upheld by the white plantocracy. By the 1960s, these simultaneous themes of conservative respectability and radicalism took center stage in Black middle-class attempts to prove their readiness for self-government, independence, and fundamental citizenship.[52] Once seen to possess the social, moral, and cultural capital fit to rule, the Black middle class, fortified with sociocultural instruction on respectable citizenship, went on to assert their place as leaders of nationalist parties in the transition toward independence from the 1960s in places like Jamaica, Trinidad and Tobago, Barbados, and the Bahamas.[53] In turn, competent leadership and nationalist rhetoric across much of the anglophone Caribbean came to be characterized by a simultaneous denouncement of imperialism and inequality and an upholding of the Victorian values of morality, respectability, and the surveillance of working-class Black femininity and sexuality. Thus came to be the biopolitical nationalist project of making the working-class Black woman respectable—tinged with compounding suspicions and pathologies around Black women's hypersexuality that would continue to haunt postindependence rhetoric and biopolitical interventions in the anglophone Caribbean well into the twenty-first century.[54]

Indeed, while much was gained with Barbadian independence in 1966, these long-standing colonial and Enlightenment discourses of rationality, cherished heteropatriarchal gender roles, and relations remained central to the functioning of the postcolonial state, which repeatedly reinscribed sexual control of Black women's bodies. Turning its back on colonial welfare policy in favor of neocolonial ideals of development, the new postcolonial state moved swiftly toward capitalist modernization under the leadership of Errol Barrow's Democratic Labour Party. Yet, as Aaron Kamugisha emphasizes, by the mid-1970s, after radical political ideologies failed to mobilize change, "the rise of an even more predatory neoliberal globalization . . . meant that the postcolonial elite's dream of equality of nation states and its liberal ideal of the equality of citizens within Caribbean nation states look[ed] more like a nightmare than anything else."[55]

Risk and HPV Vaccination in Twenty-First-Century Barbados

As discussed in chapter 1, through the 1980s, the widespread retreat of the postcolonial state from nation-building and manufacturing resulted in a widespread embrace of neoliberal globalization, its structural adjustment programs, and regional partnerships across the anglophone Caribbean. The Barbadian government's unique Social Partners model, instituted in the 1990s, made great strides in revolutionizing access to education and supporting economic growth through alliances with the private sector and nongovernmental institutions. Created in lieu of International Monetary Fund measures, this model was critical to forging a sense of civic trust in the Barbadian public into the twenty-first century.[56] Over the course of the following two decades, however, regional challenges in the CARICOM, rapid technological changes, and ongoing socioeconomic decline in the wake of the 2008 global financial crisis greatly compromised this unity, threatening the model's achievements and reactivating a sense of suspicion and government mistrust for many citizens. From the increasing immersion and precarity of Barbados in CARICOM's single market and economy program and the influx of intraregional nationals it facilitated to the growing government interest in enhancing technological development and multinational involvement across the sectors of health, border security, education, and finance, the sense of disillusionment among Barbadians toward governmental initiatives was palpable across my numerous visits to the island between 2015 and 2018.

Many whom I interviewed about the HPV vaccine questioned the financial motives behind the state's involvement in this conjoined industry–state biopolitical endeavor. Referencing colonial tropes and suspicions of Black women's hypersexuality and gesturing to the various forms of surveillance, regulation, and monitoring of Black women's bodies outlined herein, Afro-Barbadian parents often framed their suspicions alongside the shifting motivations, tactics, and factors that have historically motivated state-led biopolitical projects in Barbados and the anglophone Caribbean in the name of capitalist development. Connecting contemporary neoliberal imperatives, historical colonial violence, and the atypical promotion of the HPV vaccine, parents like Natty and Danielle further underscored how the risks of HPV in Barbados appear to disproportionately attach to Black women's sexuality. By indexing longer histories of biomedical surveillance, pharmaceutical experimentation, and profit of and on Black women's bodies, their suspicions about the HPV vaccine trace the persistence of industry, race/racism, health, and capital in risk's ambit. Naming, discrediting, and at the same time entertaining claims that both Big Pharma and the Barbadian state held the potential to harm especially the most vulnerable (lower-class, Black) Barbadians, they struggle to delineate where the health interests of their Black daughters lie amid these shifting and sometimes opposing factors, emphasizing the multiple constitutions and understandings of risk that surround HPV and the HPV vaccine in contemporary Barbados.

That public opposition to population-based risk assessment, medical technologies like vaccines, a preference for individualized knowledge, and care for oneself is a growing problem for modern medicine globally points to a notable and widespread ambivalent relationship among factors such as risk, identity, morality, and care as they converge around the practice of vaccination. Like all (bio)technologies, vaccines are *pharmakons*, fundamentally and irreducibly ambivalent—poison, remedy, or both—and often scapegoats for a plethora of societal problems, values, and understandings about health, morality, risk, responsibility, and care.[57] Asha Persson has mobilized the term *pharmakon* to explore the inherent ambivalence of biomedical drugs and technologies and particularly the polarizing nature of antiretroviral drugs and their "capacity to be *beneficial and detrimental to the same person at the same time.*"[58] Anne Pollock has relatedly explored the pharmakon as a metaphor for a specific racialized drug that is both cure and poison—with equal possibilities to treat heart failure for African Americans, alleviate health disparities, and lead to toxicity, "harm to the cause of antiracism in medicine and society, and that of profits for amoral drug companies at the expense of suffering patients."[59]

Insofar as public health discourses surrounding vaccination are often oriented toward a scientific logic of risk reduction as the basis for care and medical intervention, they effectively obscure these tensions between risk and care. In so doing, they overlook the fundamental ambivalence of vaccines inherent in claims to/of care and their frequent intersections with industry and for-profit corporations. Such ambivalences within and between care and risk are amplified in contemporary biopolitical public health campaigns in favor of the HPV vaccine, which further articulate the population risk logic of vaccination with that of sex/uality, morality, and gender.[60] Scholars Connell and Hunt point to an increasing "interconnection between moral discourse and risk discourse" through which accepting the scientific, public health, and pharmaceutical risk-managing strategy/technology of the HPV vaccine becomes doubly tasked as a moral imperative to intervene in the sexuality of young women (in particular) to whom the vaccine was initially marketed to prevent cervical cancer.[61] As this chapter has shown, these confluences take on special significance in the context of postcolonial Barbados, within whose history risk logics and medical logics have notoriously coincided in colonial biopolitics and the surveillance and control of *Black* women's sexuality from the period of slavery. These entanglements continue to manifest themselves across the manifold promotional efforts around Gardasil and in the suspicion and deliberation about the same by many of the Afro-Barbadian parents with whom I spoke.

If we return again to the Gyn-A-Thon promotional flyer (figure 2.1), it is apparent how these overlapping (and sometimes conflicting) logics and ideologies circulate in the same social media post. Simultaneously aiming to raise awareness about HPV and destigmatize it by highlighting its ubiquitous nature across sex, the flyer details the ease with which the virus is transmitted, its connection with genital warts, and implications in multiple forms of cancer. Despite this, several indications suggest that the risks of HPV attach disproportionately to women. As aforementioned, most notable of these is the striking image of a white woman's abdomen, caressed by her hands in the shape of a heart. Presumably gesturing toward an appreciation of or effort to protect her reproductive organs in the fight against HPV and cervical cancer, this image carries particular understandings of care, responsibility, and, we might say, respectability.

As I reflected on this flyer, I was reminded of a conversation with an older Afro-Barbadian woman who approached me one evening as I stood outside a local shopping complex, posting recruitment flyers for interview participants. Though she said she had no time to be interviewed, she wanted to let me know that she was a former nurse trained in England who understood the science behind vaccines. Still, she was deeply unsettled at the politics of race at play in the local promotion of Gardasil. In addition to the prominent Barbadian-born Indian doctor who was often on TV discussing the vaccine, she complained, the Ministry of Health had solicited the assistance of a white doctor from another country to help promote the vaccine. Questioning why there weren't more people like "us" leading the campaign, she wondered what message this was sending to Afro-Barbadians. Uncomfortable with how it was being promoted by these health officials, she advised her daughter against accepting the vaccine for her preteen granddaughter. Likely referring to Barbados's Gyn-A-Thon head doctor, Vikash Chatrani, and Dr. Godfrey Xuereb, the PAHO/WHO representative for Barbados and the Eastern Caribbean, she succinctly points to the optics of non-Afro Barbadians promoting this vaccine to a populace that is more than 90 percent Black. For her, such promotion coupled with a lack of transparency was a recipe for leading educated people like herself to entertain conspiracy theories about pharmaceutical companies and governments testing their new products on young Black women. Here, as with this Gyn-A-Thon Instagram post, representation matters. Beyond it probably being an ineffective form of advertising mismatched with its target audience, this flyer, like Afro-Barbadians' suspicion toward the HPV vaccine and the Ministry of Health's various promotional tactics, ought to be read in Barbados's legacy of often injurious necro/biopolitical projects and policies—especially as they relate to women's sexuality. As Afro-Barbadian parents like Natty and Danielle remind us, concerns about the vaccine and the way it is locally promoted and advertised are indelibly informed by the past as much as the current economic climate. Indeed, in a historical context of colonial violence within which Black women were deemed risky, fungible commodities and Black women's sexuality consistently subject to surveillance, management, and study, suspicion or hesitancy toward such risk logics and biopolitical initiatives ought not always necessarily be deemed conspiratorial.

Conclusion

This chapter sought to emphasize the connections between a range of colonial biopolitical projects, risk, race, gender, and capital accumulation in Barbados and the anglophone Caribbean from the eighteenth to the twenty-first century. Beginning with a history of risk assessment and its increasing use in biomedicine, it has traced the ways biopolitical projects in Barbados were rationalized by colonial suspicions toward the risks of prescribed wayward, contaminated, immoral, and hypersexual colonized peoples, centering to a considerable extent on Black women's bodies and their sexuality.

From the eighteenth through the twentieth century, medicoscientific conceptualizations of racial difference dominated imperial ideology. Variously validating abuse, neglect, and the use of biopolitics to establish a healthy and fertile labor force who would exploit raw materials in the aim of capital accumulation, resulting policies sought to physically regulate Afro-Caribbean women's bodies, control their purported natural inclinations toward hypersexuality, and save them from immorality. These frequently harmful biopolitical projects and their fixations on Black women's sexuality have historically entwined with conflictual class, economic, and political dynamics that undoubtedly implicate, but often transgressed race. In addition to white elite suspicions around hyperfecundity and hypersexuality, for example, a different but related set of suspicions around race and sexuality become apparent for the rising Black middle class, who were hoping to assume their place as nationalist leaders before independence.[62] Here it was specifically the working-class Black woman's sexuality that was in need of regulation into civility and respectability by educated middle class Black men and women in the name of nation-building. By the turn of the twenty-first century, like many other societies, Barbados was facing rapid globalization, reflected in the increased commercialization, foreign investment, and technological development in many sectors, including that of public health.

The twenty-first-century introduction of the HPV vaccine campaign in Barbados reflects a biopolitical endeavor that is historically produced and organized across racialized and classed lines and shifting socioeconomic alliances and that is mediated through contemporary technological, media, and biomedical developments. Tracing some of these key historical shifts through the conflictual and multiscaled legacies of risk, biomedicine, care, and capitalism in Barbados and the wider Caribbean confronts us with how the present continues to touch the past, its often injurious biopolitical interests in caring for and saving lives, and its multiple and sticky suspicions. In the next chapter, I specifically examine how some of these suspicions around Black women's hypersexuality sustain themselves as residue, but also how they are acknowledged, denied, negotiated, and technologically mediated under and within neoliberal globalization in Barbados today.

THREE

(Hyper)Sexuality, Respectability, and the Language of Suspicion

Raquel is an eighteen-year-old Afro-Barbadian and the first teenager I interviewed in 2015 about her views on the HPV vaccine and Barbadians' hesitancy toward it. When asked why she thought many Barbadian parents were refusing the vaccine for their children, she confidently claimed, "It all has to do with sex!" Emphasizing the taboo nature of sex and anything related to the topic in her household, she dramatically said, "I can't bring up something like this vaccine with my mother, not at all! At all, at all, at all! My mother, she's very . . . she's very closed off and boxed up. So for her anything about sex is taboo and won't leave her lips, she will just think it and be like, 'Ohh, it's my daughter, I can't speak of those things, she's just a child!'" Though Raquel was beyond the age at which the Ministry of Health was offering the HPV vaccine to students preparing to enter secondary school, teenagers like herself were still eligible to receive the vaccine at their local polyclinics. Throughout our interview, Raquel expressed great interest in the vaccine and frustration at what she believed would be her mother's objection to this idea on account of the vaccine's "sex element": "My mother doesn't want me with boys or anything like that so . . . I know that's the first thing that would come to her mind with this vaccine. And well, that's the only thing that would make her hesitant, but I will try to educate her because I would definitely get the vaccine if it was up to me alone."

Chelsea, a nineteen-year-old, similarly speculated that many Barbadian parents' resistance to the vaccine was rooted in concerns about sex. "I think it has more to do with the . . . I don't want to say image it would have, but what perceptions would come along with having your child vaccinated from the standpoint of other people judging the choices they made as parents." Reflecting on the stigmas she believed might attach to parents who accepted the vaccine, Chelsea felt that in an "image-oriented society," such as Barbados's, decisions like whether to vaccinate one's daughter for a sexually transmitted disease are under intense scrutiny. "When everybody knows everybody, you can't really get away with doing anything without someone else seeing," she explained. In her opinion, parents were likely to base their decision on the HPV vaccine "on what [their] next-door neighbor is going to think of [them] if they found out. Because for people here, it's a really big issue, just the whole idea of sex and image. . . . Yeah, it bothers people a lot, a lot, a lot what other people are going to hear or find out about them."

Chelsea's and Raquel's confident theorizations about Barbadian parents' suspicions and refusals toward the HPV vaccine were not dissimilar from those of the medical practitioners with whom I spoke. Like these teenagers, the doctors and public health nurses I interviewed unanimously claimed that it was parents' concerns about sex, their children's sexual activity, and a "cultural" adherence to a politics of respectability that were the predominant drivers of suspicion toward the HPV vaccine. Although public health officials often adamantly claimed that fears about respectability were the primary motivators of resistance to the vaccine, less than 10 percent of the parents I interviewed supported these beliefs. Following the seemingly contradictory articulations and theorizations of suspicion toward the HPV vaccine by Barbadian medical practitioners, Afro-Barbadian adolescents, and parents, this chapter details the multiple ways (hyper)sexuality, gendered norms, and affects around sex and technology come to frame concerns around the HPV vaccine, to highlight how suspicion is complexly entangled with (rather than indicative of) an adherence to colonial narratives of respectability. Guided by adolescents' reflective commentary on the multiple silences and suspicions that surround their sexual bodies, it further explores how smartphones and social media platforms are, like the HPV vaccine, similarly vectors for the circulation of suspicion in Barbados—one that extends from adolescents' sexual bodies to these technologies and the Barbadian state.

The notion of respectability emerged in eighteenth-century Europe amid white bourgeois concerns around "'decent and correct' manners and morals, as well as the proper attitude toward sexuality"—cultural ideologies and behaviors that quickly became subsumed and sanctioned by European nationalism.[1] Typical markers of respectability, including education, heterosexual and holy matrimony, regular church attendance, and nuclear households, first made their way to the Caribbean during slavery via the planter classes and were reinforced through missionaries' attempts to institute social order, civility, and Christianity in colonial society through the postemancipation period.[2]

As noted in chapter 2, as nationalism rose across the 1960s anglophone Caribbean, Black men and women of the rising middle class sought to uphold values of respectability through education and training by the British on proper modes of conduct, citizenship, and moral rectitude, hoping this would distance them from the stereotypes of irresponsible working-class masculinity and promiscuous female sexuality and establish themselves as elevated citizens with the virtues deemed necessary to self-govern.[3] As in the United States, which saw reverberations of these respectable ideals in its middle-class Black communities, adoptions of these politics by Black, middle-class anglophone Caribbean leaders only amplified underlying class and gendered tensions among Afro-Caribbeans who actively resisted the ideals of respectability despite their shared goal of freeing themselves of colonial rule and moving toward nation-building. Indeed, by no means universally adapted, a plethora of Caribbean scholarship has detailed how many Afro-Caribbean people rejected notions of respectability in the postemancipation Caribbean by maintaining traditional social norms and actively protesting against respectability's racist and classist premises, which were fundamentally at odds with long-standing social norms like matrifocality in many creole Caribbean communities.[4] Such works relay the nuanced modes of resistance, livability, and expression that Afro-Caribbean women specifically engaged in from the abolition of slavery through the postemancipation period, accounts that run counter to what is often described as a prescriptive and inescapable legacy of respectability for Afro-Caribbean women.

Chief among proponents of claims to such a legacy of respectability is anthropologist Peter Wilson, who argued that a widespread adherence to respectability politics could clearly be observed among Afro-Caribbean women from the postemancipation period and into the postindependence era.[5] This respectability, he argued, existed alongside a distinctly competing and gendered value system of reputation. Within this paradigm of respectability/reputation, Wilson claimed that Afro-Caribbean women were lured by the European value of respectability rooted in whiteness, heteropatriarchy, colonial order, and sexual modesty, whereas Black men were more concerned with the masculinist value systems of reputation—described as an anticolonial, countercultural, nonelitist, and indigenous to African culture.

Caribbean feminists have repeatedly challenged Wilson's deeply controversial text, *Crab Antics: The Social Anthropology of English-Speaking Negro Societies of the Caribbean*, in which he forwards these arguments, offering important revisions to its reductionist, gendered paradigm and overwhelming emphasis on normative families and heteronormativity.[6] Despite significant critiques and evidence of distinctly creole value systems, state-recognized informal conjugal relationships, a widespread body of theorization on nonheteronormative Caribbean sexualities in the postindependence anglophone Caribbean, and the indisputably contradictory ways bourgeois values of respectability and moral sexual conduct have translated to different classes of Afro-Caribbean citizens after independence, politics such as those Wilson outlined remain persistently influential among academics in labeling respectability as an ideal to which Afro-Caribbean women especially ascribe. As Carla Freeman notes, in scholarship on Afro-Caribbean peoples, "most [theorists] find it impossible to dispense entirely with the idea of a central dialectic," resulting in a retention of these value systems as the "locus or expression of Caribbean cultural authenticity."[7] Although respectability politics have been widely criticized by Caribbeanists, Vanessa Agard-Jones further argues, they continue to be drawn on in response to narrative prescriptions of Caribbean people as hypersexual.[8] As Faith Smith notes, norms of colonially influenced respectable sexual conduct continue to inform the "structures of feeling of the region's peoples" regarding morality and sexuality in everyday life in the Caribbean.[9]

Indeed, the tenable parameters and silences around sex and sexuality are well reflected in the puritanical approach to the topic of sex across much of the Caribbean. Frequently disguised in secrecy and shame, talk of sex is often relegated to the realms of music, theater, and innuendo.[10] At the same time, the language of sex has unmistakably, consistently, and hypervisibly framed social and cultural life in the region in ways that challenge and resist a politics of respectability and heteropatriarchy.[11] What are we to make of these contradictions and dualities in and around respectability politics in the Caribbean and in Caribbean scholarship? This chapter takes this question as a starting point to explore the language of suspicion and its relationship to colonial narratives of respectability.

All of the immunization nurses with whom I spoke across Barbados's nine polyclinics believed that concerns about sex were largely to blame for parents' hesitance to accept the HPV vaccine for their daughters. According to Nurse Browne:

> I think that it's a culture thing . . . because you know we got this perception that a girl can get pregnant so easily but we don't realize it's the boy who is impregnating her so once it comes to anything to do with se[x], you always got a barrier where the girl is concerned, right. The boys can have the vaccine because there's the view that, "Look, a boy will be a boy and if he becomes sexually active then he's covered. But a girl now you don't want to expose her to sex." The mere fact that a vaccine makes her mind open to sex, to being involved with sex [makes] it a big no.

Much like the teenagers with whom I spoke, professionals like Nurse Browne believed parents' concerns reflected the pervasive societal and cultural attitudes in the Caribbean around sex, specifically women's sex and sexuality. My interviews with parents, however, provided a range of generative perspectives from which to complicate teenagers' and nurses' popular understandings of parents' preoccupation with respectability and premature female adolescent sex. Unfaithful to popular understandings of their refusal of the HPV vaccine as embedded in a politics of respectability, Afro-Barbadian parents overwhelmingly described their suspicion as complexly fashioned by a multitude of layered and cross-temporal concerns and legacies.

When I expressed confusion at the diverging understandings about vaccine refusal and suspicion between nurses and parents, Nurse Brant insisted:

> Although they didn't say it in so many words, many parents were concerned that their daughter would go have sex with John, Jack, and George. So objectively I can say that they were concerned simultaneously about the harm it could have on the children, the potential side effects, and too, the sex factor.
>
> . . .
>
> There's a lot of concern at the root of it, especially surrounding girls and sex. They don't want them to have sex. One father came in with his twin children, one was a girl and one was a boy. And he consented to the vaccine for his son, but not his daughter. So we saw this. We saw parents, even some fathers, being protective and saying no.

For Nurse Brant, though parents might not have expressed an outright concern about their daughters engaging in premature sexual activity, their differential attitude toward the vaccine for their sons was enough of an indication that their concerns transcended the side effects they might have also claimed to be concerned about. If not for a concern around women's sexuality, she argued, why would such a parent accept the vaccine for his thirteen-year-old son but not his twin daughter? Nurse Parker, an immunization nurse from another polyclinic in southwest Barbados, reiterated many of Nurse Brant's thoughts, stating, "I don't think parents want to talk about it, that's the truth, right? But I mean, when you look at how the parents of the boys seem to be so accepting it really shows you that it has something to do with the concern about these girls, these 'angels' versus the guys, right? Nobody wants to consider their ten-year-old daughter having sex." Nurse Parker speaks to the politics of silence around female adolescent sexuality and to what she perceived to be the cultural acceptance of (adolescent) male sexual activity in light of many parents' differential willingness to vaccinate their sons. Although both nurses comment on the perceived ease with which parents accepted the vaccine for their sons once it became available to boys in 2015, they also conceded that it was impossible to say with certainty whether parents' reactions would have been the same had the vaccine been offered to boys during the program's initial roll-out in schools in 2014. Nevertheless, nurses maintained the belief that it was the Barbadian "culture" around sex that was affecting parents' beliefs about the necessity of the vaccine for boys and the inappropriateness of the vaccine (and sexual activity) for adolescent girls. As another nurse commented to me, "In our culture, it's okay for boys to have sex but not girls, so this is all probably part of the difference in uptake."

I couldn't help but notice the irony in that parents' perceived forms of silence and concern around sex and sexuality were reflected in nurses' silences of the same. As was evident during the vaccine's introduction stage in the United States in the early to mid-2000s, when the vaccine was first introduced in Barbados in 2014 we find the simultaneous appearance of persistent attempts by medical professionals to circumvent discussion about the risks of HPV as they relate to sexual activity and to advertise the vaccine as a cervical cancer preventative vaccine. As the Ministry of Health expanded its market to Barbadian boys in 2015, we find another related trend, whereby discussion of anal cancer is widely avoided by medical professionals (for fear of [homo]sexualizing the vaccine) and through which the advertised benefits of the vaccine to Barbadian parents of young men and women largely focus on protection against genital warts and cervical cancer, respectively. Although talk of genital warts and the protection against cervical cancer in boys' (female) sexual partners did occasionally occur, none of the Barbadian nurses or practitioners with whom I spoke mentioned anal sex or the protection the vaccine provides against this and other sexually transmitted cancers in men when discussing the HPV vaccine. Perhaps this is indicative of their own biases and taboos around sex and homosexuality, even as they critiqued parents for their perceived concerns. This obfuscation of the risks of HPV for Barbadian boys and men and its connections to anal, penile, and head and neck cancers is both noteworthy and unsurprising. As Mamo and Epstein note regarding the US context, such a "careful management of sexuality" within the marketing and discussion of Gardasil strategically deflects attention from the connections between HPV, sex and sexual transmission, and attempts to submerge the ever-looming reality that men who have sex with men are at significantly higher risk of contracting HPV.[12] Beyond these striking omissions and blanket statements about perceived parental anxieties around sex, these and other nurses make significant claims about the gendered disparities implicated in parents' suspicions of the vaccine that are worth further investigation.

As M. Jacqui Alexander notes, such invocations about gender, culture, and sexuality are intimately connected to race, socioeconomic status, and nationalism—categories that, like morality and respectability, are socially constructed.[13] Indeed, partly through the socially constructed gendered dynamic of respectability might we explain the ease with which a father weighs his decision making about the HPV vaccine for his twins. His decision to accept the vaccine for his son can arguably be said to be guided by a belief that he is in the public sphere and driven by reputation; conversely, the resistance he expressed toward vaccination for his daughter could hypothetically be guided by notions of respectability. Yet a closer engagement with Caribbean feminist literature on gendered ideologies and the masculinist policing of women's sexuality on the part of the state and its male citizenry complicates this neat reading of respectability as underlying hesitancy toward the HPV vaccine for Barbadian girls. Caribbean feminist V. Eudine Barriteau has theorized extensively on the inescapability of Caribbean gender relations and societal expectations to which many nurses referred, noting how cultural, economic, and political dimensions of gender interact in public domains with significant material and ideological effects.[14] As Barriteau notes, both "material and ideological relations of gender are relations of power."[15] Although material relations dictate gendered access to (and distribution of) resources in society, ideological relations of gender shape society's understanding of femininity and masculinity: "[They] indicat[e] how a society's notion of masculinity and femininity are constructed and maintained. The ways in which [they] are constructed reveal the gender ideologies operating in a state and society. . . . The social expectations and the personal constructions of gender identities form the core of gender ideologies within a particular society."[16] Caribbeanists have further stressed the influence not just of patriarchy but processes of heterosexualization on these ideologies and the neocolonial state formation in the anglophone Caribbean as a whole, such that gender and sexuality are culturally normalized and actively regulated by the state.[17] This process occurs through a number of tactics such as policies that silence sexuality and laws that differently construe and construct citizens based on their gender and sexual practices. Emphasizing the anglophone Caribbean state's multifaceted nature, these Caribbeanists detail its existence as a web of relations with power that is neither singular nor centralized but ever shifting and emerging across a number of institutions. As Barriteau notes, for example, "state power is exercised by a minister of health, and by sanitation workers cleaning the streets. The latter may daily extend the boundaries of state power in areas unknown both to the public and to ministers who may assume they alone define the scope of that power."[18] That the biotechnology of the HPV vaccine was initially introduced on behalf of the state to intervene in women's health in a context in which there are striking gendered health differentials (partly due to the region's gender norms) is arguably a progressive move for heteropatriarchal states such as Barbados, Guyana, and Trinidad and Tobago, the latter of which preceded Barbados in introducing the vaccine to young girls through a national program in 2013. Yet as Barriteau reminds us, societal boundaries establishing gendered relations of power are often nuanced such that a "Caribbean society may permit women to take on responsibilities essentially constructed as masculine, as long as these do not produce a corresponding shift in gendered [or other socially constructed] relations of power," including sexuality and religion.[19] A close examination of the HPV vaccine campaign's rollout and reception in Barbados ought not lose sight of the state's multiple arms, its various allegiances, and roles in consolidating and upholding these relations of power.

Building on Alexander, Latoya Lazarus discusses the centrality of Christianity to nationalist projects in twenty-first-century Jamaica.[20] Insisting that we recognize its influence as deeply embedded in the foundation of the anglophone Caribbean state, Lazarus notes that "the nation is continuously being gendered and sexualized in ways that support and normalize a heteropatriarchal discourse and structuring principle."[21] Christianity, she emphasizes, works to shape "people's attitudes towards sexuality and sex-related issues," across the citizenry, from parents and politicians and public health practitioners.[22] The 2013 temporary suspension of the HPV vaccination campaign in Trinidad and Tobago is a case in point. The suspension arose after the Catholic Education Board of Management opposed administering the vaccine to young girls in its primary and secondary schools. The board argued that it was not properly informed of the program's initiative and its merits in advance of its initiation and called for an immediate suspension and consultation. Although the program was reinstated after the requested consultation, this example reinforces Lazarus's claims regarding the centrality of Christianity to the workings of the anglophone Caribbean state, even and especially during cases where state institutions like the Ministry of Health depart from the heteropatriarchal status quo to introduce what was perceived to be an explicitly gendered and sexualized technology.

Whereas Barbados's decision to initially introduce its HPV vaccine campaign exclusively to young girls followed international models, the widespread marketing of Gardasil as a cervical cancer vaccine to target young women's risk of contracting HPV prior to the initiation of (heterosexual) sex unsurprisingly invited the circulation of cultural understandings and ideologies of gender that questioned the vaccine's "appropriateness" for the adolescent girls to whom it was targeted. When the ministry extended the vaccination program to boys in 2015, nurses claimed that parents overwhelmingly accepted the vaccine for their sons. Doing so, we might say, predictably follows the heteropatriarchal hierarchy created by the anglophone state, which prioritizes and even celebrates men's heterosexuality and its risks. Thus, while this one father's acceptance of the vaccine for his son and refusal for his daughter might be framed in a politics of reputation or respectability, it is also likely constituted by and constitutive of well-established gendered ideologies of the anglophone Caribbean state whereby women's sexuality, sex, and its risks are policed by masculinity. To wholly conflate or subsume such narratives in a reputation/respectability paradigm loses sight of these more insidious and nuanced gendered ideologies at play and the similarly complex understandings of both respectability and Caribbean gendered ideologies parents brought to their elaborations about suspicion. As I argue in this chapter, nurses' claims about parents' hesitancy too neatly and often uncritically frame suspicion of the vaccine in a presumed politics of respectability and desire to silence a discussion of adolescent sex, eliding the powerful lineage of colonial anxieties around Black women's hypersexuality and heteropatriarchy through which parents overwhelmingly articulated the affective feelings that surrounded the HPV vaccine.

When asked directly how they would respond to parents' suspicions about the vaccine and potential concerns that it might encourage their daughters to engage in sex, nurses described the importance of stating the facts about HPV and its ubiquitous transmission via skin-to-skin contact and emphasized the need to reassure parents of their mutual aims to protect their children rather than encouraging them to engage in sexual activity. Nurse Alleyne served as part of the Ministry of Health's vaccination team in 2014 and was responsible for co-facilitating town hall meetings, seminars, and lectures on the HPV vaccine at parent-teacher association meetings in secondary schools. Speaking about the ambivalence she observed from parents who were concerned about their daughters having sex, she notes:

> Some parents had this mindset that giving the girls the HPV vaccine will cause them to want to have sex. [But] you know how it is [*laughs*]. The boys can do no wrong. And you hear things like, "I don't want my girls having sex" and "If you give the girls the HPV vaccine it will give them license to have sex." We had to say to them, "Listen, some of these girls have been having sex for years now, HPV vaccine or not. What we are trying to do is prevent them from long-term problems down the line." But parents were saying, "But why [do] I have to give it to my daughter, my daughter is not even sexually active?" . . . So I would smile inwardly because these parents are standing so confidently telling me that their daughters were not having sex, but as a nurse I know differently.

Others mentioned parents' underlying concerns over the impression that accepting the HPV vaccine would have in a rigidly socially stratified society such as Barbados. Like Chelsea, some nurses argued that Barbados's small size caused citizens' desires to adhere to a politics of respectability to be all the more acute. According to Nurse Parker, beyond personal concerns about the vaccine representing a license for children to engage in sex, parents were preoccupied with thinking about what other parents would believe or what insinuations would be made about their daughters and their sexual behavior if they were to receive the vaccine. She described how parents would sit together in polyclinic waiting rooms while their children received routine booster shots to enter secondary school, casually chatting but also closely observing each other's decision making about the newly offered HPV vaccine. The effect that certain upper-middle-class, (often white) parents had on many other lower-class parents, she suggested, could not be overlooked: "Parents are in the waiting area all together and they kind of talking and looking, you know, so it's that kind of influence. Like, so, 'Okay, she saying no and she brighter than me and well off and if she's not giving it to her child then I'm not either.' On the other hand, if that person is saying, 'Okay, I'm letting my child have it because of xyz,' we see how that would affect others too, you know?" In addition to suggesting that parents were concerned about what other Barbadians might insinuate, comments like Nurse Parker's elucidate the classed and racial tenets presumed to inhere in parents' hesitations to accept the vaccine, whether or not they are framed in a language of respectability. As mentioned in chapter 2, for a number of self-described middle-class Afro-Barbadians, their various positionalities vis-à-vis the state, level of education, and keen perceptiveness of the processes of gendered, sexualized, and racialized pharmaceuticalization that surrounded the vaccine's introduction to Barbados all factored into their decision making.

As one middle-class Afro-Barbadian mother named Alicia described to me, outside the realm of respectability politics, careful consideration of the vaccine and monitoring of the decisions of other parents were especially warranted with something like the HPV vaccine. For Alicia, this was just one of many examples reflecting the unnecessary imposition of state and foreign interests, medical techniques, and decisions onto Barbadians. Because it was parents' responsibility to protect their children from abuse and manipulation by "the powers that be," she felt, refusing this vaccine should be viewed as an educated decision that she and other Barbadians were more than capable of making, despite the country's small size:

> You know, we need to get people to understand that together, we can fight. I think that society and even [as a region] we can stand together and not be guinea pigs because that's what we are setting up ourselves to be if we just accept [this vaccine]. And people think that we don't have the financial wherewithal, we don't have a voice, and that gets under my skin. Sometimes Bajans are very passive. . . . Does the Ministry of Health perhaps think that they can push this because Bajans will just be accepting of it? Passive is not the same as uneducated. . . . Bajans are very educated.

Another Afro-Barbadian mother, Denise, felt that her suspicions and ultimate decision to refuse the vaccine were "smart." When many citizens were disillusioned with the Barbadian government, being skeptical about its most recent marketing scheme, its underlying aims in disseminating the vaccine, and paying attention to who accepts and who does not, she argued, was logical and prudent. For Denise, careful consideration of the vaccine and the decisions of others was especially warranted because the HPV vaccine represented pharmaceutical interests and government imposition.

Such explanations for suspicions about the vaccine differ significantly from nurses' confidently articulated beliefs about parents' suspicions. While many Afro-Barbadian parents might uphold gendered ideologies and values of respectable conduct and comportment, nurses largely foreclosed other possibilities for parents' ambivalence to the vaccine, instead ubiquitously attributing suspicion to concerns about adolescent girls' sexuality and a presumed adherence to a postcolonial, national politics of respectability. In the following pages, I continue to read interviews with Afro-Barbadian parents who expressed suspicion about the vaccine to more accurately reveal the constitutive ambiguities of their suspicion and highlight the multifaceted ways these parents simultaneously refuse, deny, and sometimes perpetuate claims to respectability politics around women's sexuality and hypersexuality. I detail how these parents' collective invocations of respectability in their discussions of suspicion largely depart from nurses' claims and from contested scholarly understandings of the widespread turn to a politics of respectability among Afro-Caribbeans.

Complicating Respectability through Suspicion

Bee is a thirty-nine-year-old Afro-Barbadian mother of four and part-time sales associate who refused the vaccine for her daughter. Bee described her family's approach to biomedicine as "contentious" on account of the chronic health issues she had been facing over the past fifteen years and her belief that pharmaceutical drugs and "chemicals" were largely to blame. "I have sickle cell trait and I have my blood valve prolapse and between the two of those things, God knows what else. I have been weak and listless and everything else for so many years and umm, I realize that you know, I don't really have to feel like this. If there is a certain way that I can eat or some things and some drugs that I can avoid to help me feel better, then I will [do that]." During our conversation, she described how the online research she had conducted over the past few years provided her with a different perspective on pharmaceuticals, which she now resorts to only if the situation is dire, in favor of organic foods and natural or herbal remedies. Given this context, she expressed great concern over the potential side effects of the HPV vaccine on her ten-year-old daughter and the lack of assistance she and her family would receive from the government should these potential side effects be severe and long-lasting.

Although all four of her children received childhood immunizations, Bee felt differently about the HPV vaccine. When asked if concerns about adolescent sexual activity played into her decision making, she shook her head and said:

BEE: No, no. Because me, well when I came up sex wasn't even a word in my house. I got my period at twelve and [my mother] told me . . . this is going to happen to you every month unless you do something with a boy and then it's gonna stop. I didn't know what I was going to do with a boy [laughs]. . . . Well, my daughter now, she started hers at only nine. . . . When I told my mother she started, she was surprised, and she told me to tell her all the different things that she never told me [laughs] but at ten? She doesn't need to know that at ten years old! She has to know how to position the pad in her clothes so they don't dirty . . . that is what she has to know.

NICOLE: Okay, so is it that you don't think it's time to talk to your daughter about sex yet? You don't think it's appropriate?

BEE: No. If, when she is exposed to [sex], say, in secondary school, I will have to let her know not to let boys get too close to her, not to let nobody touch her in a certain way. She will have to know that from the time she steps into secondary school for sure, but I think if you raise a girl to respect herself, if you live your life decent, then . . . Look, she only see me in here with her father. Anybody that I hugging up go be a close friend, or my brothers or my father, and I ain't go do with them like how I do with their father and they ain't go see me do much with their father [*laughs*]. So it's going to be a whole respectful kind of upbringing. She will learn to respect herself from young, and protect herself too. . . . I think that children might turn to that sort of a lifestyle to fill a gap. Your father ain't there, or he don't like you, or he don't treat you good, or you don't get fed properly or whatever that will send you out to look around for other people to fill this space in your life.

While Bee jokes about the lack of important information about sex and pregnancy she received from her mother when she began to menstruate, she appears to be repeating this history as she shares a reluctance to talk to her adolescent daughter about these issues. Bee's comments about modesty and respectable behavior suggest that if her daughter adheres to the forms of modesty that she teaches and models then she could avoid "*that* sort of lifestyle"—one she seems to think might necessitate the HPV vaccine. When I asked her to elaborate on the lifestyle she referred to, she responded:

So as long as I think you give the child everything it needs . . . everything, nurture the whole child, everything . . . not just food but teachings, then she will be happy where she is . . . and she will respect herself and know how to protect and defend herself too from these things and diseases, and that's about how I see it. I mean, I know I can't just say "that kind of lifestyle" because you can be harassed, you can be assaulted . . . but there are ways you can minimize being exposed to this type of thing.

Though she gestured "no" in response to my initial question about whether her decision to refuse the vaccine was in any way connected to concerns about adolescent sexual activity, there is a consistent slippage in her language around lifestyle, sexual behavior, and desire. Framing a lifestyle of promiscuous or premature sexual activity as a void one might choose to fill to seek happiness, Bee suggests that nurturing and providing for her daughter and teaching and modeling respectable behavior would bring her happiness and ultimately protect her from the risks of sex and sexually transmitted diseases such as HPV, thus potentially negating the need for this vaccine.

Views like Bee's draw attention to the importance some Afro-Barbadian parents might place on upholding and modeling a politics of respectability for their children in the ways many nurses seemed to suggest. Yet the contradictions in Bee's comments intrigued me—relics of which were present across several of my interviews with parents who refused the vaccine for their children. Like Bee, when asked directly if they had concerns about the vaccine's relationship to sex and sexual activity, most parents denied that their suspicions were rooted in anxieties about adolescent sexuality or respectability. At the same time, these parents consistently invoked themes of modesty, respectable behavior, and adolescent sex in their discussions of suspicion. Yet, as I detail shortly, rather than simply advocating for respectability as a protective quality that could ameliorate the need for the HPV vaccine as Bee does, parents' comments overwhelmingly reflect the nuances of respectability politics and make powerful claims about how middle-class Afro-Barbadians are negotiating gendered ideologies and colonial narratives of hypersexuality, which high rates of sexually transmitted diseases (STDs), teenage pregnancy, and cervical cancer in the Caribbean all seem to suggest, allude to, and create suspicion around.

For instance, when I asked Pamela, an Afro-Barbadian writer and mother of two children, whether she had concerns about the vaccine's association with sex, she responded by framing her suspicions around the vaccine's side-effects: "Nobody has convinced me yet why it is relevant to give a ten-year-old, eleven-year-old, twelve-year-old the human papillomavirus vaccine . . . putting that in her system at such a young age. . . . It's not there now, and I don't know if in the future if it would affect her body when she gets to be an adult." Insinuating that her eleven- and twelve-year-old daughters were not yet sexually active, Pamela was both suspicious about the need to expose them to HPV antibodies so early in their lives and worried about the long-term effects the vaccine could have on her daughters in the future. Her argument about exposing her daughters to the vaccine "at such a young age" was one I heard from several parents and was especially problematic for medical practitioners seeking to increase compliance toward the vaccine, since the rationale for targeting eleven- and twelve-year-old children is based on scientific evidence that indicates increased efficacy if introduced prior to the initiation of sexual contact. Although Pamela began by framing her suspicions around the vaccine's side effects, our conversation did eventually turn to sex:

> Because they were saying, I guess what [the nurses] was saying was that umm, if the child is promiscuous too, then it's important . . . and that's the thing that have me. This idea of the girls as promiscuous. If you raise your daughter . . . Yes, you can't, you can't predict the future, but if you're raising your child to have morals and standards and stuff like that then I don't know if my daughter needs this right away. But yes, I know there is a high prevalence of sexual activities in secondary schools now too. So . . . well . . . I just don't think that is up to me to put that HPV in her system when it's not there now.

Like Bee, Pamela suggests that a promiscuous lifestyle is synonymous with adolescent sexual activity in and of itself. Though she incorrectly conflates the two, what she largely appears to struggle with is the idea that her daughters could be sexually active as early as secondary school. She oscillates between a discomfort with the narrative that her daughters are promiscuous—suggesting that she raises her daughters according to a prescribed set of respectable values—and the defeated recognition that secondary school children of her daughters' ages are in fact engaged in sexual activity in Barbados. The contradictions in Pamela's statements at once reveal her belief that modesty, morality, and proper sexual comportment could prevent her daughters from being labeled promiscuous (and potentially prevent them from contracting HPV) and that her suspicion is, to a significant extent, about the prescribed labeling of her Black, preteen daughters as sexually promiscuous and in need of this vaccine. In arguing, "that's the thing that have me," Pamela asserts that this characterization of promiscuity, one that reverberates colonial stereotypes, is what is so deeply unsettling.

David, a forty-nine-year-old Afro-Barbadian, schoolteacher, and father of two mentioned in chapter 1, also refused the vaccine for his daughter, Daphne. His articulations of his suspicions extend and elaborate those expressed by Pamela. In our interview, although David acknowledged the potential benefits of the vaccine considering the prevalence of cervical cancer in places such as Barbados and the developing world, he framed his ambivalence around his skepticism toward the multinational pharmaceutical industry behind its manufacturing. As he noted, "It's not that we never administer drugs to our children, but this particular one though, nah. Two hundred million vaccines, US$150 per shot . . . Big Pharma is mekking a lot of money out of this thing!" While David conceded that he did associate the vaccine with sex, he claimed that he was not concerned about it encouraging his daughter to engage in sexual activity. Although he was personally uncomfortable talking about sex with his twelve-year-old daughter, he acknowledged the importance of doing so and the reality of teenage sex, and he described being no stranger to the range of pertinent questions adolescents have about their bodies and sex because of his job as a high school teacher. Rather, like Pamela, David felt that marketing a vaccine (one that protects against an STD) to Barbadians such as his daughter evoked disturbing colonial stereotypes of Black women's hypersexuality.

This process of pharmaceuticalization, or the collision of multiple local, state, corporate, and nongovernmental organizations and actors with the workings of the pharmaceutical industry, is an increasingly global phenomenon that facilitates the "transform[ation] [of] the right to health into the right to treatment (including prevention) with pharmaceuticals."[23] In their comparative study of the HPV and hepatitis B vaccine (which prevents liver cancers), Mamo and Epstein further note how processes of pharmaceuticalization surrounding Gardasil in the United States have occurred alongside processes of sexualization wherein risks around HPV and sex are constructed through the vaccine's development and broader sociopolitical logics.[24] As explored in chapter 2, sexual risks and practices come to be categorized in Barbados around and in relationship to the HPV vaccine, its enmeshment in socioeconomic and political contexts, and longer injurious histories of colonialism. Here we might further note the extent to which these risks are produced through scientific and pharmaceutical claims about gender, risk, and sexuality such that it is predominantly young Afro-Barbadian women who become the targets of the state-pharmaceutical nexus's intervention (rather than the disease of HPV itself), and vaccination comes to signal prevention, responsibility, and the "right to health."[25]

David felt that officials promoting immunization were under the belief that Black women in the Caribbean were "highly sexed" and in need of help and protection through this vaccine. In conveying his wariness about such designations, David proclaimed himself to be a pan-Africanist who was well attuned to persistent colonial tropes about Black women's hypersexuality and critical of how the promotion of the vaccine enabled such ideologies to thrive. Beyond an identity, pan-Africanism speaks to the ideological belief in a shared history and collective future for peoples of African descent on the continent and across the diaspora.[26] By invoking these phenomena, David situates his suspicion within a legacy of revolutionary mobilization among Black peoples transnationally against slavery and colonialism, persistent racisms, and economic, political, and sociocultural forms of oppression within which he situates the HPV vaccine and Barbadian state–industry processes of pharmaceuticalization and biopolitics.

Simone, a middle-to-upper-class Afro-Barbadian mother, similarly framed her suspicions about the vaccine in a legacy of racist histories. As a consultant who worked in the realm of health, Simone was knowledgeable about STDs like HPV and the importance of sexual health education for girls and young women in Barbados and throughout the Caribbean. Nevertheless, she refused the vaccine for her daughter. Worried it would disconnect her from her responsibility to manage her own sexual health risks, she resented the idea of her daughter submitting herself to the control of pharmaceutical companies and their technologies. Reflecting on long-standing histories of suspicion toward Black women's bodies and the resulting surveillance, violence, and biopolitical regulations imposed on their bodies throughout the period of slavery, Simone feared that accepting the vaccine for her ten-year-old would fundamentally threaten her daughter's right to autonomy over her body and sexual health.

These parents draw associations between the vaccine and the colonial tropes of female hypersexuality and respectability politics without reducing or wholly attributing their suspicions to a concern about their children's sexual activity. Denying a simple adherence to respectability and emphasizing their knowledge about HPV and its potentially serious repercussions, David and Simone gesture instead to the vaccine's ability to disconcertingly reproduce stereotypes and pathologies around (Black) women's hypersexuality in the Caribbean. Although Pamela suggests a belief in the value of respectability, she more squarely associates her suspicion with what she felt were nurses' unsettling characterizations of adolescent girls' hypersexuality. Across these parents' articulations of suspicion, the historical antecedents for discussions of the HPV vaccine are clear. In its call to protect the adolescent female body from the risks of its sexual activity, the vaccine gestures to a range of racialized histories around sexuality and population control in Barbados and the wider Caribbean. These are histories and biopolitical tactics of which Black women's bodies and their supposedly uncontrolled sexualities were—and are—the target and Black women the figures on which risk continues to be attached.[27]

For Pamela, David, Simone, and other Afro-Barbadians with whom I spoke, these narratives of hypersexuality and the vaccine to which they attach themselves generate suspicion. Here, suspicion around the vaccine and its connections to female adolescent sexuality should not be wholeheartedly conflated with parents' simplistic adherence to respectability or concerns about what others might perceive about their daughters' sexual activity. Instead, these interviews suggest that many of these middle-class Afro-Barbadian parents' suspicions reflect a much more complex recognition of hegemonic colonial stereotypes of Black women's hypersexuality and a desire to protect their children from these psychic, palimpsestic residues and harms. Such comments further gesture to a distrust of the Barbadian government and the neoliberal global circuits of technoscience, ethics, economics, and pharmaceutical exchange of which the vaccine is a part. Indeed, beyond expressing conservatism around sexuality and a belief in the protective potential of a politics of respectability, even Bee—who rationalized her rejection of the vaccine in terms of respectable conduct—connects her suspicions to distrust in the government, its precarious economy, and its interests in protecting the Barbadian public. Like sex and respectability politics, the state recurs heavily in many parents' suspicion.

For instance, some struggled to reconcile the intense promotion of this vaccine (initially exclusively targeted toward young girls) with what they perceived to be the heteropatriarchal state's more mundane, strategic, and misaligned priorities when it came to the sexual health of adolescents. Female adolescents' inability to access contraceptives without parental consent was an example of one such policy mentioned by one Afro-Barbadian mother and hairdresser named Selena. Although the age of consent for sexual activity in Barbados is sixteen years, adolescents below the age of eighteen cannot access sexual and reproductive health services and treatment without parental consent because they are considered minors under the Barbadian Minors Act.[28] Although there are no laws preventing adolescents from accessing these services, they are unable to secure birth control pills or information on other contraceptives, safe sex, and STDs in government clinics or pharmacies unless they have their parents' support and accompaniment. Despite no specific legal mandate being in place here, the state's nebulous categorization of adolescents between the ages of sixteen and eighteen holds control over their sexual intimacy, rights, and risks and restricts female adolescents' independent access to prescription contraceptives. As some of the teenagers with whom I spoke noted, these unmet sexual and reproductive health needs, along with a lack of comprehensive sexual education in schools, are partly to blame for the high rates of teenage pregnancy and HIV/AIDS among their peers today.

Referencing this disparity in the law as a basis to question not the appropriateness but the necessity of the vaccine, Selena questioned the urgency with which ten- and eleven-year-old girls were being offered the vaccine by the government when under its same rule they weren't able to access contraceptive pills until eighteen years of age. Frustrated, she wondered, "What are the government's real priorities when it comes to adolescent sex and sexual health? Why the forceful promotion of technologies like the vaccine to preteens yet the intentional restrictions around sexual health in other regards?" Tying her suspicions about the vaccine to what she deemed an atypical biopolitical campaign, Selena reinforces the fact that postcolonial relations of gender ought to be understood not only in terms of a colonial legacy but as "features of civic and political life" that are sustained by state systems precisely for how they "satisfy specific, indigenously defined objectives of state interests."[29] Indeed, even as states try to act with citizens' best interests at heart, as Barriteau notes, "policies implemented by governments may reproduce existing gender asymmetries, they may intensify, decrease or subvert them, but policies are not gender neutral."[30] Knitting together these realities, Selena contextualizes suspicion toward the vaccine within her relationship to the heteropatriarchal state's asymmetric intervention into female adolescent health amid a lack of gendered access to important sexual health material resources.

David also supported these assertions, arguing that the government's stated goal to save lives with this vaccine inevitably occurred alongside its efforts to fulfill economic allegiances and partnerships with multinational pharmaceutical companies like Merck and the biomedical technologies they manufacture. This was amid the increasing precarity of the Barbadian state, its economy, and the financial security of the Barbadian public. Regardless of its (un)stated aims, both capital gain and life optimization are likely satisfied in the successful marketing of the HPV vaccine to the Barbadian public. As David incisively recognizes, the state's provision of life-saving technologies to the public should not distract us from its shrewd enmeshment in for-profit pharmaceutical assemblages, which necessarily capitalize on the risks of adolescent girls' (sexual) health by marketing technologies like the HPV vaccine. Drawing attention to wider transnational biopolitical, technoscientific networks, or "global assemblages" of exchange in which the Barbadian state has immersed itself since the 1980s and which have become increasingly technologically oriented, David invites us to consider how suspicion sticks to and extends to these mushrooming networks, expanding pharmaceutical industries, public–private partnerships, and their respective technologies and policies that connect with broader global configurations of power.[31] As a rich field of anthropology has also explored, beyond biotechnologies, a growing range of communication and information technologies play an increasingly central role in mediating and transforming national and transnational economics, intimacies, and affects like suspicion.[32] Echoing these truths, many of the adolescents I interviewed drew connections between technologies like the HPV vaccine and their smartphones—technologies that, like the HPV vaccine, attracted unwanted attention to adolescent sexuality. The following section examines these connections in closer detail.

In September 2016, the Barbadian government introduced a new cellphone policy to replace an almost decade-long ban on cellphone usage in schools. The new plan acknowledged the use of smartphones and other information technologies as valuable learning aides, outlined guidelines for their responsible use in primary and secondary schools, and reiterated the government's plan to invest BBD$2 million to retool schools with tablets, laptops, and computers under the Education Sector Enhancement Programme.[33] Prior to the introduction of this policy, which coincided with my first research trip to Barbados in 2015, the issue of devices in schools was one of contentious debate among citizens. From my survey of newspaper articles and editorial commentaries, interview discussions, and informal conversations with the general public, citizens acknowledged the benefits of these technologies for educational purposes and underscored the importance of Barbadians staying ahead of the digital revolution that has been occurring in the region over the past few years. Many also expressed resistance to the use of smartphones in schools, concerned at the frequency with which they were being used by students to engage in cyberbullying, pornography, and the sharing and recording of sex in schools. Such concerns were not without precedent.

In October 2013, Barbados's major newspaper, the *Nation News*, posted a story headlined "Sex Scene," along with images of two fourteen-year-old minors engaging in sex in an empty school classroom. Three newspaper employees were arrested and charged under Barbados's Protection of Children Act for the inappropriate posting of this material, but the swarm of public debate around the incident focused on the adolescents' lack of morality and respectability, their lewd behavior, and the importance of abstinence-only education.[34] As Corey Worrell, former Commonwealth Youth Ambassador, commented, "I say this to the young people: sex is amazing, but the irresponsible and ungodly use of a penis and vagina will destroy your life. Condoms protect your flesh but don't protect your heart or your soul, so they aren't completely safe, but abstinence is."[35] Yet there is nothing novel about this scandal, its portrayal by the media, or the reaction to it from the Barbadian public. Unfortunately, the cultural disrespect for data privacy and lack of journalistic integrity have been well documented throughout the Caribbean over the past decade, evident each time another of these adolescent sex scandals occurs.

Another such incident occurred in October 2014, when two homemade videos of students from St. Rose's High School in Guyana surfaced online. Viral on social media sites within hours, the videos purportedly show the young teenage students clothed in school uniforms and engaging in oral and penetrative sex while smiling into the camera, suggesting an awareness of being recorded. One week after the videos appeared online, the state-owned *Guyana Chronicle* newspaper printed a front-page photograph of two of the students engaged in sex with their faces clearly visible and another larger image on an additional page. While Priya Manickchand, Guyana's Minister of Education at the time, expressed outrage at the *Chronicle's* unprofessional journalistic work and called for parents, schools, and churches to engage adolescents in a more open dialogue about sex, the public's reaction was overwhelmingly one of condemnation and stigmatization toward teens, with comments such as "Deal with them and don't let them off the hook lightly" and "Take them out of school.... [They] are ... destroying the school systems."[36] As with the incident in Barbados, school officials' responses further elicited themes of disappointment and anxiety around the nation's moral decay. For instance, St. Rose's High School arranged for motivational speakers to host guidance seminars at the school both to "set [students] back on track after the shock release of [the] video" and assure concerned citizens that steps were being taken to restore pride to the high school that is often touted as one of the most prestigious in the country.[37]

Exhuming panic, such comments frame adolescent sex as a serious moral problem. Its widely proposed public remedy forgoes teaching teens about safe and responsible sex in lieu of preaching the benefits of abstinence to restore and keep intact the moral values of Caribbean schools and societies that are continually being tainted in light of such scandals. In my interviews with Afro-Barbadian adolescents, many criticized their parents and school boards for failing to provide this information, claiming that sex in schools was common and ignoring it was to remain willfully ignorant of the need for sexual health education. In the wake of the aforementioned media publicity around sex and smartphones in secondary schools, teenagers shared their assertive beliefs about the suspicion that underlay smartphones, their sexual activity, and the elusive HPV vaccine.

I began my interview with a group of four eighteen-year-old boys at an all-boys secondary school by trying to gauge their knowledge about HPV and the newly available HPV vaccine. Amid giggles and teasing, all four confessed to little knowledge about the virus besides its sexual transmission. They quickly steered the conversation toward HIV/AIDS, syphilis, and the clap (gonorrhea), the more well-known STDs, which they indicated they frequently discussed and harbored concerns about:

PAUL: You should learn [about how to protect yourself] in school, because like, this is an everyday thing. If these diseases are spread every day and it's as rampant as they say, then we should really have more information on them.

DARRYL: Yeah, educate us so we know what to do and not to do instead of saying, "Say no to sex," because we going to have sex.

NICOLE: So where do you go to for information if not in school? The internet? Your parents?

RYAN: Parents, no way. I guess friends mainly, but you get more pressure than advice from friends to just do it, and older siblings, too. I even got teased from my father when I entered secondary school that I was still a virgin.

BRIAN: Yeah, peer pressure. In primary school it would start like, "Oh, I can't believe you never got anything yet," and by secondary school if you don't have sex by now then you are nobody.

NICOLE: And so, do you think girls face this same pressure?

DARRYL: There is a different standard because say you are a girl child, your parents will try to protect you from the world, and not tease you about not having a boyfriend.

RYAN: But girls still do it though. It's a way to relieve stress. Girls our age and younger do it all the time, in schools and all.

NICOLE: Is sex in schools a very common occurrence apart from what is publicized in the newspapers?

RYAN: Hey, it's an everyday thing. It's an everyday thing.

DARRYL: In the school I used to go to . . . it used to happen every day and it ain't only happen between kids, it happens between kids and teachers.

RYAN: Check it, it's not only that it's the heat of the moment, but it's the only time we get. Some people don't get time to actually go anywhere with the person and such so they say well, we here now, let we go and take it.

BRIAN: Even in primary schools you hear about some children doing it, all nine and ten years old because they getting exposed to the sex from early.

Together, these comments express the boys' interest in gaining education about sex and STDs but also insinuate that societal pressures for them to lose their virginity are perhaps more urgent than seeking information on safe sex and STDs. While they expressed that the Barbadian government and its school systems generally fail to provide comprehensive sexual health education, these same schools serve as convenient (and often the only) places for teens to have sex.

When I inquired about their views on the recent debates around allowing cellphones in schools and parents' hesitations about these technologies, these and other teenagers argued that parents' anxieties around smartphones and apps like Snapchat were in fact misplaced concerns about adolescent sex, something they claimed has always occurred among people their age:

NICOLE: Do you agree that teens are using technologies for the wrong purposes in schools?

DARRYL: They could be. Yes and no. You see, back in the day, things with sex were the same; it's just like people didn't use to record it and such. But listen, technology still helps us because don't forget we use it to do our schoolwork. ... What we need to do is educate the youth on how to use technology in the schools instead of just saying no. Because really and truly all of these things that are happening now were happening back in the day. Like when my father was a youngster, he was telling me about stories that happened in his time and he is near fifty. It's just that social media now is bringing it to the forefront.

For Darryl and others, suspicion over technologies from smartphones to the HPV vaccine is amplified due to the ways they call attention to sex and necessitate that the reality of adolescent sex be reckoned with.

Raquel similarly felt that suspicion around cellphones in schools was a failed attempt to mask societal anxieties around teenage sex. In denial of the reality of teenage sex, she noted, her parents and the Ministry of Education were failing to provide her and her peers with sexual health education and knowledge about STDs such as HPV:

RAQUEL: The problem is we just don't learn about these things. Okay, we have a guidance counselor . . . but that was not effective at all. I swear that woman was so boring and she has a million things to do. Out of a term of twelve weeks I would have seen her like three times. . . . We had one class that dealt with sex about the sexual organs, but like it was not effective at all. I remember one time our physics teacher took over her class and he had . . . two papers, a blue and a pink one and he stuck them together and then he tore them apart and he like, asked the class, "Y'all see what happened there?" The pink paper had some blue pieces and the blue one had some pink stuff on it . . . [so] he drew an analogy to sex because when you have sex, he said you retain some of each other. And that was the lesson.

NICOLE: And was the lesson helpful for you?

RAQUEL: It was kind of was a scare tactic . . . but it's not helpful because schoolchildren are having sex. . . . Last week . . . a teacher walked in and saw two students having sex. And I don't know where you can do it at [this school]. . . . The school is so open, so open. . . . People tell me the art room, and I'm just like, "No . . . no, no, no, no. You mean the art room where they had to clean because they found a rat?"

NICOLE: And is this happening at other schools, too, you think?

RAQUEL: Oh yes, it can become a culture at school. I remember there was a little acronym: SALT [sex at lunch time]. . . . Yeah I can remember some videos I saw of students doing oral and having sex at schools. And that's happening in lots of schools. Queen's College (QC) is another school that's "up there" in terms of ranks but I would say that it's too much of a pride thing for it to get out that QC students are doing that too even though they are. But I would say that like Springer, Springer is one of the lower schools and it's always getting out these videos of them and then it go viral then and it might even be a one-off situation but because it's a video now it's like, "Ohhh this always happening, the children is the worst!"

NICOLE: And what do you think is influencing this trend of sex in schools?

RAQUEL: Well me, I eh know what to think. I think a lot of people is just assuming . . . assuming with this "trend" because umm, back then it probably was the same in terms of how much sex or how many people were having sex. . . . I mean, back then I don have no statistics but . . .

Beyond reiterating the male teenagers' beliefs in the ubiquitous nature of adolescent sex, Raquel's comments emphasize how the suspicion that surrounds the use of smartphones and laptops in schools, like the suspicion surrounding the HPV vaccine, is entangled with class. She makes astute observations about the class politics that exist in the suspicion around sex and the acknowledgment of the prevalence of adolescent sex. As a student at one of the island's most prestigious high schools, she draws connections between other esteemed schools where sex among students and parents' suspicions of the same are supposedly less frequent only because of their lack of publicization. Teenage sex throughout schools of varying status, she hypothesizes, has long existed.

Courtnee, a seventeen-year-old Afro-Barbadian who attended the same school as Raquel, similarly explained to me that the anxiety around technologies like cellphones in schools was, at its core, suspicion over adolescent sex and its optics. "Before there were iPads, there were cell phones, and before that there were cameras, so I don't think it's that technology is the problem to be banned. And I think it's an exaggeration when the media says teens are out of control; that might only be a subset, a select few. They are saying that we are out of control, so sexually active, but, I'm seventeen and I haven't had sexual intercourse." Indeed, as reiterated by Darryl, Courtnee, and Raquel, although sex at lunchtime has an acronym that can be texted and sexual acts can be recorded and shared via smartphones, teen sex in school or elsewhere is in no way a new phenomenon. Such claims insist that we acknowledge the unspectacular nature of adolescent sex and how suspicions around it have long existed in the Caribbean. What is novel is the introduction of technologies that intervene on and make viral adolescent sex. Suspicion attaches to these technologies in part for their ability to resurface discourses of excessive hypersexuality—discourses that are problematic not only for Afro-Barbadian parents but, as it appears, for Black middle-class young women like Courtnee, who attend prestigious schools and adamantly resist the media's characterizations of themselves as uncontrollable and irresponsible young women who have sex in school.

Following these teenagers' claims, we might think of these suspicions around smartphones and this invocation and speculation of respectability politics as a response by Barbadian citizens to the country's turbulent economy, the weakened nation-state, and growing suspicions around its former government's shifting allegiances and widening assemblages of multinational corporations in the realm of health care and beyond. To be sure, school sex scandals and the comments that surround them foreground the relationship between sex and technologies and the proliferation of these technologies under neoliberal globalization, whereby adolescent sex and the technologies to which it is connected come to represent much of what is wrong and superfluous in contemporary Caribbean societies.

As with the HPV vaccine, filming and virtually sharing teen sex with smartphones and laptops in schools surface a range of suspicions around these technologies and their facilitation by the Barbadian and other anglophone Caribbean states. Front and center, adolescent sex becomes fixated on, not only as something spectacular or morally disturbing but as a troublesome indication of increasingly vulnerable and weak nation-states struggling to maintain political power yet unable to control their optics, their citizens, and their schools. As David Murray has argued, technologies like cellphones and the sexual activity they highlight function as figurative ghosts for citizens' pertinent anxieties over many of Barbados's socioeconomic and political ills, including its precarious economy, lowering levels of tourism, political subordination, a withdrawn government, increasing unemployment, and the region's increasing marginalization at the global level.[38] Although the amplifications in use and discussion of technologies (and suspicions toward them) in the realm of sexuality and public health are by no means unique to Barbados (and are perhaps even mundane throughout much of the developed world today), the effects of these processes are context specific.[39]

There is something particular and potentially transformative about the effect of a proliferating range of global biomedical and communication technologies on adolescent sex in a place like Barbados, where social structure and affective memories have been indelibly affected by a system of plantation slavery and the postcolonial state has long regulated sexuality and citizenship through the use of very measured "technologies of control," which are critical to its reproduction.[40] As I have illustrated throughout this chapter, in addition to and beyond nurses' beliefs that parents' suspicions of the HPV vaccine were driven by a faithfulness to respectability politics, Afro-Barbadian parents' suspicions attach to teen sex, to the perception of hypersexuality, and to the many technologies, spatiotemporal conditions, arrangements, and economies that are impossibly entangled in sex's mediation in postcolonial Barbados. Emphasizing suspicion's residual, affective nature, Afro-Barbadian parents' narration of suspicion toward the HPV vaccine points to its diffusive tendencies and its historical lineage, rendering it powerful and lasting but also divisive. For their adolescent children, suspicion attaches to them as parents and to the state, both perceived to misplace their suspicions and attention on technologies that mediate, illuminate, alter, and enhance adolescent sex in lieu of sexual health information.

Conclusion

One enters a room and history follows; one enters a room and history precedes. History is already seated in the chair in the empty room when one arrives. Where one stands in a society seems always related to this historical experience. Where one can be observed is relative to that history. All human effort seems to emanate from this door. How do I know this? Only by self-observation, only by looking. Only by feeling. Only by being a part, sitting in the room with history.
—DIONNE BRAND, *A Map to the Door of No Return* (2001)

Dionne Brand's prescient words invite us to consider the complex histories through which belonging, being, and existence have been constructed for people of the African diaspora.[41] The histories to which Brand refers are palimpsestic, with layers of trauma, sexual subjection, and violence under slavery punctuating, conjoining, and lingering as residue with and within Black people's contemporary lived histories of racism and refusal.[42] These histories, Brand argues, cannot be let off the hook, for they affect and reflect the contradictory tropes, suspicions, and experiences informing diasporic identity today.

This chapter explored the languages through which suspicion around the HPV vaccine is spoken and spoken about in Barbados by medical professionals, adolescents, and Afro-Barbadian parents with whom I spoke. Following adolescents' thoughts on parents' respectability politics, and reflecting on the tropes of hypersexuality and the subsequent silences and suspicions around sex that have for so long come to define the Caribbean and its citizens' relationship to sex, I began to lay out some of the contradictions and ambiguities that exist for Afro-Barbadian parents as they experience and negotiate the colonial provenance of hypersexuality in connection to the adolescent girl's body and the HPV vaccine. Although a rich legacy of research has spoken to the threats that the homosexual body poses to heteropatriarchal nationalist frameworks in Caribbean nation-states, less attention has been paid to the roles that adolescents similarly play in upholding the state's fragile heteropatriarchal values and the subsequent fractures their sexualized bodies pose to nationalist constructs and citizens' relationships and identities.[43]

As my interview excerpts with Barbadian nurses and parents reveal, suspicion toward or refusal of this technology appears to be as much about the unsettling, racialized, and gendered hypersexual activity it brings into focus as it is about affective memories and residues of the control, denigration, and hypersexual tropes enforced on Black women under slavery and in postcolonial bio/necropolitical regimes that cannot be let go of. For many Afro-Barbadian parents, the government's questionable ruses and involvement in pharmaceuticalization processes complicate and constitute a multiplicity of suspicions around the state and proliferating global technologies from smartphones to laptops.[44] The angst in Caribbean citizens' newspaper comments over adolescent sex scandals involving smart devices in schools is just one example of the broad range of concerns these suspicions encompass. As parents like David, Bee, and Selena uniquely express, apart from a wariness about adolescent immorality and (dis)respectability, the government's decision to promote this vaccine in the way it did and at the expense of seemingly more urgent forms of support and care further surfaced Barbadian parents' deep-seated anxieties over a sense of their nation's decay—both moral and economic in an era of rapid socioeconomic change and restructuring of transnational economic, pharmaceutical, and political alliances in the Caribbean. Refusing a retrenchment into respectability politics, the parents herein overwhelmingly present the tensions implicit in the lived reality of respectability and hypersexuality in the Caribbean.

In presenting some of these tensions as they coalesce around technologies like the HPV vaccine and long-standing ideologies of gender in the anglophone Caribbean, I also aimed to foreshadow how these technologies and the affects they stimulate foster divides and relationships between differently situated citizens in Barbadian society. Afro-Barbadian parents' suspicion has much to offer us as Caribbean feminist, humanities, social science, and technoscience researchers as we wrestle with colonial inheritances, their disturbing reflection in neoliberal state processes and narratives, and the messy implications of these entanglements for the health and protection of our region's citizens. Chapter 4 looks to this issue of protection and suspicion as a powerfully fraught embodiment of care and defense.

FOUR

Care, Embodiment, and Sensed Protection

VERSION A

Nurse. Parent. Teenager. Vaccine. Cold. Fluid. Vial. Dilute. Swirl. Syringe. Needle. Sharp. Distract. Quick. Puncture. Skin. Penetrate. Flesh. Tissue. Pain. Infiltrate. System. Redness. Swelling. Time. Surveillance. Repeat. Protection.

VERSION B

Nurse. Parent. Teenager. Vaccine. Media. Pharmaceuticals. Money. Suspicion. Internet. Research. Community. Videos. Surveillance. Memory. Flesh. Pain. Force. Skin. Reproduction. Fear. Gut. Feeling. Unknown. Consider. Reconsider. Refusal. Protection.

In an interview with a well-known Barbadian pediatrician about parents' hesitancy toward the HPV vaccine, Dr. Jones said to me: "I think after a while, people will come to their senses, do what's best and protect [their children]." To which senses do we refer when we speak of "coming to one's senses"? I wondered. For Bernadette, a thirty-nine-year-old Afro-Barbadian mother of two, coming to her senses meant reasoning through her deepest feelings of suspicion and doubt to refuse the HPV vaccine for her twelve-year-old daughter: "It's very difficult when you have a child and you're trying to see what's the best thing for their health, protection, for their lives, you know? It's really daunting, but I felt, I feel really convicted in what my deep instincts were." Whereas Dr. Jones invokes a sensibility whereby one acts according to biomedical knowledge and instruction to protect the body from disease, Bernadette articulates an instinctual sense of suspicion to similarly protect her daughter. Version A and version B collide.

Like Bernadette, many parents with whom I spoke expressed a suspicion that engendered both skepticism and an impulse to protect. For these parents, suspicion was a form of protection—a visceral sense through which HPV vaccination is framed as antithetical to protection. How does suspicion inhere in, constitute, or impede protection? What might it mean to "come to one's senses and protect," as Dr. Jones claims, if we consider the multiple meanings of the word *sense* and the material and psychic histories that, like palimpsests, inform Barbadian parents' suspicion toward the HPV vaccine?

According to the *Oxford English Dictionary*, the word *sense* carries multiple meanings.[1] A sense, we might say, is a capacity through which the body recognizes a stimulus, a feeling, or intuitive awareness to the presence of something, or the way an event can be interpreted. Sense, as in good or bad sense, also describes a mode of discernment, while *to* sense or to perceive by sense is to attune to the reality of something without a clear articulation of how one comes to that knowledge or realization. Occupying claims to rationality, the phrase "to come to one's senses" more specifically suggests restoring one's consciousness after some period of irrationality. Likewise, to have or to be in one's senses—to be sensible—is to be sane and in full control of one's thoughts, words, and actions. But sensibility might also be thought of, in the words of self-defined Black lesbian feminist mother poet warrior Audre Lorde, as "a disciplined attention to the true meaning of 'it feels right to me,'" that is, an instinctual feeling in and through the body—a form of mindedness through which reason and protection are achieved.[2] Eschewing the conflation of sensibility with rationality, such a consideration of sense more capaciously recognizes sensing as the body's ability to detect or feel stimuli that are enfleshed: from pain and temperature to visceral senses like memory and affects like suspicion.

This chapter considers these various constitutions of the word *sense* and its derivative, *sensibility*, within, as, and in response to suspicion. Interrogating the contradictory understandings of care and protection emerging from these various attachments to sense and sensibility, it wrestles with the simultaneously generative and fraught nature of suspicion and its presumed protectiveness for Afro-Barbadian parents.

When you are out here in the diaspora every day, you get to know the pulse of the community and how they think and so on, and then we know how to deal with them, how to meet them at their level and get them to . . . you know . . . Without deceiving them, we tell them the truth, but there's something called too much information sometimes, so you just don't volunteer [it] because it won't make *sense*. —NURSE ALLEYNE

Darcy is a thirty-seven-year-old Afro-Barbadian homemaker and mother of two daughters. She expressed uncertainty over vaccinating her eldest daughter, Paula, with the HPV vaccine. In our interview, Darcy said her ambivalence was motivated by fear of the vaccine's side effects and the aggression she perceived to accompany its promotion. After her two-year-old daughter suffered multiple traumatic seizures and emergency hospital visits after receiving some routine childhood immunizations, Darcy made the difficult decision to forgo her remaining vaccines. Though thirteen-year-old Paula responded normally to these same vaccines, Darcy feared the stress and pain from her recent experiences with her youngest were too intense to imagine bearing again, even just for one vaccine. Recognizing the potential benefits of the HPV vaccine, Darcy reiterated that she and her husband were still considering it yet were also very concerned about the forceful way the Ministry of Health was presenting the vaccine to Barbadian parents:

> The nurses and doctors in Barbados . . . they had a program that was on TV recently and these nurses were trying to like, forcefully push [the vaccine]. . . . She was like, "You have to get the vaccination, it is a must" and "If you don't, you know, this will happen and that will happen," and someone called in and said, "Well, are there alternative methods to the vaccination that you could try like homeopathic medicine?" And she just shut that down and said, "No, that is not safe, and it's not proven." To me it was just like, "Just get the vaccination, just get it . . . no questions asked." And it seemed like they were trying to just push it down and force it down your throat without parents having an opinion about it. Yes, yes, and that pushing made me uneasy you know, like disturbed.

Darcy describes the manner in which public health professionals impose vaccination on parents not simply in ideological terms but in physical terms, likening nurses' pushiness to a forceful imposition on and through the body. Sensing this force alongside a perceived disregard for her concerns about the vaccine, she calls attention to the viscerally charged nature of force and suspicion and the unsettlement and unease they engender. I was struck by Darcy's use of the phrase "force it down your throat," variations of which I noted several parents used to refer not only to the government's efforts to promote vaccination but to its proposed introduction of policies and technologies like biometric screening machines, discussed in chapter 1. Conjuring the perception of aggression and power that such biopolitical initiatives contained, this phrase indexes the democratic state's enmeshment in burgeoning global assemblages in which citizens are deemed fortunate and passive beneficiaries of their biopolitical techniques, technologies, and promissory modes of a protection. With respect to vaccination specifically, it materializes the physicality of the vaccine; its sharp components; its unpleasant, painful insertion into the body; and its public health administrators working urgently on behalf of the state to instill that pain and force, if only temporarily and in the name of protection.

For Denise, the thirty-nine-year-old Afro-Barbadian mother mentioned in chapter 3, the insistent promotion of the vaccine was one of many examples that she felt reflected the unnecessary imposition of pharmaceutical products on Black people:

> I think that we Black people are so umm, we are brain, we are brainwashed to believe in things even when we can't even see the common sense in it. We don look for the common sense in it. We don't look to put two and three together. We let someone come and push something down we throat all the time and say, "Oh, yeah, yeah, it's fine." Mm hmmm. We don't sit down and analyze. We don analyze. We does just say yeah, they want us to get that—no problem. And then we go ahead with it. No! They are only now having a vaccine for this [HPV]. This thing has been around for ages and they are now having a vaccine for it? So what I believe is that now they are rat testing us people. No!

Denise is not only wary that Afro-Barbadians will uncritically accept the vaccine because of the government's forceful promotion but concerned at the limited time frame in which she felt the vaccine had been tested. Suspicious that she and other Afro-Barbadians had become test subjects, she gestures to the longue durée of scientific and medical study and intervention on Black bodies under slavery and the colonial period and to more recent histories of medical experimentation on people of color and their sexual health across the African diaspora throughout the twentieth century, which were underlined by force, coercion, and deceit. From the targeting of poor, uneducated, disenfranchised Puerto Rican women as experimental subjects in birth control trials of the 1950s to the duplicitous recruitment of ailing Black men into Tuskegee syphilis experiments under the guise of medical care from the 1930s to the early 1970s, suspicion toward the intent of biomedical intervention among Black populations is not without reason and precedent.[3] Like Denise, Danielle and Natty (mentioned in chapter 2) referenced these histories by name, connecting affective memories of these racialized pasts to their present experiences of suspicion, distrust, and skepticism around the HPV vaccine in hopes of protecting their daughters from psychic traumas.

Since at least the 1970s, women of color feminist theorists have emphasized the power of embodied emotions and intensities like suspicion, pointing to the histories from which they emerge as "fus[ing] together to create a politic born out of necessity," that is, a "theory in the flesh" guided by the "physical realities of [the] lives [of women of color] — [their] skin color, the land or concrete [they] grew up on, [their] sexual longings," and the multiple contradictions and confluences within these lived experiences.[4] Grounding the struggle for knowledge in the body, a theory in and of the flesh embraces flesh as a guiding force, disrupting traditional Western epistemologies of sensibility as equivalent to rationality. As theory in the flesh, suspicion names and appreciates Afro-Barbadian parents' sensed feelings of unease and the epistemologies of protection they produce. Following and reasoning from these embodied senses, physical and psychic realities, mothers like Darcy and Denise gesture toward an alternate vision of protection made manifest through refusal of the vaccine and implore us to reckon with the multiple ways the knowledgeable body makes sense.

Naitry, a fifty-one-year-old mother of two daughters, similarly shared feeling resolute in her decision to decline the vaccine for her fourteen-year-old daughter, Ashley, clearly grounding this knowledge in her body. "Give it to her as soon as it reaches Barbados, have it done," she remembered her doctor advising about the HPV vaccine prior to its introduction through the national program. Naitry was similarly warmly encouraged to seek out the vaccine by family members, including her adult daughter who herself had received the vaccine in Canada, where she lived and worked at the time of our interview. Despite these trusted endorsements, years of experience making decisions for her children's health by listening to her gut ultimately informed Naitry's refusal:

NAITRY: I did a lot of general reading and research, reading articles in the newspaper and around the place, and I continuously came about articles where, you know, mothers would be saying, "Well, after my child got this vaccination she developed multiple sclerosis or you know, she had this horrible adverse reaction." In one case a parent said her child developed early menopause and wouldn't be able to bear children, and the doctor said there was no hope that they could reverse the condition. All it takes is a search on-line to the *Guardian*, the *Telegraph*, the *Post* . . .

NICOLE: And so, you did this reading and became concerned? You said that your pediatrician advised you to get it, did you talk to her about your concerns after reading what you did online?

NAITRY: I kept it to myself simply because, umm, in my experience, in my general experience as a layperson, when you tell the doctor that you're concerned they usually "pooh" your concerns and tell you that, basically, "We're the experts and we know better and you should really trust us." And I've learnt—because I'm fifty-one—I've learnt you know, that if something doesn't feel right in your gut, chances are it's not totally right, you know? And I've decided it needs further investigation and I would rather have it investigated further for a few more years than to have my daughter get it and have something happen to her. And I won't sit and have someone tell me that my concerns are invalid . . . she is ultimately my responsibility, it's my responsibility to protect her. The doctor can tell me, "Oh, go ahead" because if something happened she'd just say, "Well, it was a risk that you took and she just happened to be one of the sensitive ones." But it is *my* daughter who would have to live with the consequences.

Like Bernadette (with whom I began this chapter), Naitry relies on her gut instincts to make the decision to refuse the HPV vaccine for her daughter. Rather than describing a distrust of her doctor and the pharmaceutical company's financial interests, Naitry grounds her decision making in the fact that it is ultimately her job as a mother to protect her daughter, and thus she notes feeling compelled to follow her innermost instincts about the vaccine even after consulting with medical professionals and doing her research online. She further reveals a presumed need to protect these gut feelings from scrutiny by her daughter's doctor based on her previous experiences in which she felt they were delegitimated or overlooked in favor of evidence-based biomedical advice. For Naitry, "coming to her senses" to choose protection is reflected through an honest exploration and commitment to her sense of suspicion—to what is known, felt, and embodied—and a refusal of the unknowns that she perceived to accompany the vaccine. Audre Lorde reminds us that embodied experiences and affects like these are empowering sites of power knowledge—as much political as they are emotional. The erotic "life force" to which she speaks are "those physical, emotional, and psychic expressions of what is deepest and strongest and richest" in women of color.[5] For Lorde, this innermost sensing, feeling, and sense of feeling exists as a responsibility that women of color have for fulfillment and understanding and for scrutiny of the oppressive forces that frame our lives.[6]

Janine is an Afro-Barbadian mother of two who, like Naitry, refused the vaccine for her thirteen-year-old daughter, Sydney, by "going with her gut feeling." Sydney was offered the vaccine in 2014, at which time the Ministry of Health was still administering the vaccines in secondary schools. Janine's second child, a ten-year-old son named Paul, sat with us on her verandah as we spoke. Paul has a rare genetic and neurological disorder characterized by developmental delays, learning disabilities, and an absence of speech. Throughout our interview, she questioned her doctors' failure to detect this disorder prenatally and the prescription drugs she took during her pregnancy, which, she thought, might have affected her son's development. Consistently referring to disabilities such as Paul's as a potential side effect of this "new" HPV vaccine, Janine shared the intensity with which this challenging lived experience has framed her decision making about several medications and drugs since Paul's birth. Although she vaccinated both her children with their routine immunizations, she was skeptical about the need for the HPV vaccine on account of its then-recent entry to the Barbadian market and the sudden choice she had to make about something so unknown to her within a two-week time period in which she received and had to return the consent form to her daughter's school. When I asked how she came to the ultimate decision to refuse the vaccine, she emphasized relying on her gut:

JANINE: I asked some people at work. . . . I just asked them like, well their children are only now coming up, they are younger so I was like, "You getting the thing?" and some people are all, "Yeah, yeah man, they say it's good for [the children]." Also, before the deadline I called their pediatrician, I called [Paul's] doctor and I think I had asked my gynecologist and everybody was like, "Yeah, if it helps the girls, nothing wrong with it!" And I am like, really? I don't think so you know? So then I went to work now and asked the others again and some now were like, "I eh sure, I got to do more research," and others were like, "Yeah, they say it something good." So some people were like "No problem," and others were like, "I'm going to think about it."

NICOLE: So, after some more thought you decided no? Did you do any additional research on your own?

JANINE: Well yes but you see with this one, I am just going with my gut feeling. I am just . . . they administering it too young, it dealing with your reproductive organs, you don't know what go happen down the road. I mean yeah, you could get special needs kids without anything abnormal happening but furthermore getting that in your body and then the little research I did you hear about people fainting, swellings, and all sort of other long-term thing and I'm like, uh uh, no. And then the government pushing yuh, "Get it, get it, get it." Why you pushing it hard like that? And the minister coming on the TV and making us feel like we stupid Black people. Just lay off that!

Like Naitry, Janine sought medical advice and guidance from colleagues and friends when deciding about the vaccine for her daughter. Despite its widespread validation, she decided to refuse the vaccine based on a bad sense—an instinctual realization of discomfort and suspicion. She connects these gut sensations to similarly embodied, visceral, and material sensations and experiences of force, reproduction, and futurity. Here, she speaks to futurity in terms of protecting her child—the symbolic future of the nation—from the potential and unknown side effects of the vaccine and in terms of protecting her daughter's ability to reproduce future generations. When I asked whether she thought the vaccine could in fact protect Sydney's reproductive system by protecting her from cervical cancer, she said, "Maybe, yeah, but the area it dealing with—reproduction— that's a tricky area. Because when you offset that, you offset . . . you cutting out a whole next generation or whatever, and we, I don't wanna take that risk if something goes wrong."

This slippage between the scientific and embodied sensibility to protect reproduction is intriguing, and something I noted continually across my interviews. While many of the aforementioned parents describe doctors and nurses forcefully imposing the vaccine and its evidence-based science onto them to protect their daughters, they argue for an even more powerfully motivating inner sensibility through which their decision making about protecting their daughters' reproductive capabilities is made. Often viewed as irrational by medical professionals, these gut feelings, sensibilities, and theories in the flesh are frequently dismissed as uninformed, making parents who are suspicious about the vaccine "feel like stupid people" or feel the need to keep these gut feelings private for fear they would be ridiculed or summarily overlooked. This is true despite the scientific rationale about the role of the gut and its hormones on the body and the mind. Indeed, the nervous system controls the gut through the pituitary gland, much in the way it does the brain. Bidirectional communication, scientifically referred to as the gut-brain axis, is an important influencing factor for a plethora of human processes from adrenal function and growth to reproduction.[7] Put another way, while parents' gut sensibilities to refuse vaccination might be viewed by public health administrators as nonsensical, as feminist phenomenologist Elizabeth Wilson notes, "the gut is always minded," multiply engaged in sensing, comprehending, and ruminating.[8] When it comes to Black people (Black women specifically) and the weight that racism holds on their bodies, an acknowledgment of what feminist disability studies scholar Margaret Price calls the bodymind—the explicit and often implicit overlapping of mind and body—is crucial.[9] Theorizing this concept, Black feminist theorist Sami Schalk invites us to release our investments in mind-body dualism to better understand "the relationship of nonphysical experiences of oppression—psychic stress—and overall well-being," for people of color and their decision making about what constitutes well-being in the entangled realms of health care and biomedicine.[10] Emphasizing this imbrication of mind and body and attuning to their erotic knowledge, Afro-Barbadian parents effectively underscored the sensibility of their suspicion and its protective qualities.

Differing sensibilities of protection are illustrated through the discursive framing of the vaccine itself. As Dr. Pack, a Barbadian doctor, shared with me, "I don't call it the HPV vaccine. I call it the cancer vaccine. Because I think if you change the terminology it helps to . . . We are dealing with regular, average Joes out there. They may not be science oriented, so we need to make it simple for them and say, 'Look, this is a vaccine against cervical cancer, and that's a serious disease.'" Often referred to as the cervical cancer vaccine, the HPV vaccine protects against four strains of HPV, two of which are high-risk (cancer-causing) strains. By offering protection against cervical cancer—the second most common cancer in Barbadian women aged fifteen to forty-four—the vaccine, like suspicion does for many Afro-Barbadian parents, works to protect the female body and reproductive system. Despite Dr. Pack's belief that strategically referring to the vaccine in this way might lead "average Joes" to more easily accept it, for many of the parents with whom I spoke, attempts to desexualize the vaccine and refocus attention to the medical disease of cervical cancer failed to detract from their suspicions, particularly those around potential side effects of the vaccine on reproduction. For mothers like Janine, who frequently commented on her suspicions around her pregnancy and the relationship between the drugs she might have been prescribed and her son's disability, concerns about the vaccine's side effects on her daughter's reproductive health were especially acute. Likewise, for parents like Bee and others mentioned in chapter 3, whether the vaccine is promoted as that which targets the disease of HPV or as that which fights against cervical cancer, concerns around reproduction and the nation's futurity remained central to their suspicion.

Near the end of our interview at her home one afternoon, I asked Bee if there was anything further that she would like me to know about how she came to a decision to refuse the vaccine. Her response reiterates concerns over potential side effects and expresses a deep fear about how the vaccine could negatively affect girls' futurity in an economically precarious Barbados under the rule of a government which appeared increasingly unable to provide for its citizens:

BEE: I just wonder if they are really going to keep pushing for this thing just because it is being done in bigger countries. Because you know sometimes they does be like, "Oh, we gotta do that too." Why? You know? With something as serious as this! If you want to imitate a lil TV show, fine, I don't really care. You go out there, you get people to dress up, you sell them American clothes, whatever. But something like this, that is going to kill children, no. And it's a small little island too. For what? A death is a death and you gon fret 'bout it only when it's too late. . . . But what about the girls that you are sending, that you are literally carrying to their deaths? Because everybody is not going to make it. It's going to be all right for some people. Some people are going to be maimed and that in and of itself should tell the government who never got money, who ain't got money to support the people, it should tell them something. Because you mash up my daughter and then potentially her daughter or children too. And we ain't working for no lot of money, and now we have to come home and look after our daughters if something happens. Then [the government] got to support we, but where is the funding? If you gonna mass murder, or mass make invalids out of a lot of people, you have to have resources to fix the problem. They are going to be dropped out of the workforce. . . . They are not going to be in the workforce. And people who were in the work-force are going to be coming out to look after them! Everybody is not going to benefit. The ones who are going to benefit are the big companies, the same Merck that make the vaccine, and GlaxoSmithKline and the rest of them . . . the big boys. Nobody in Barbados is gonna benefit. So the government is going to have to look at what the repercussions are because they are going to be creating a problem. They thought they were going to be fixing a problem and protecting the girls but that's probably not going to happen, you're creating the problem. How are you going to fix that problem that you created?

NICOLE: So you're concerned that perhaps the government of Barbados is not really thinking this through fully?

BEE: They're not! And this is a small place! I mean [a] girl on [a] Facebook video I saw from New Zealand . . . she might be one of forty in New Zealand . . .

or one of two hundred in New Zealand but look how she came out. But here, well, everybody is gonna know somebody that that happened to. This is a small, small place, and you gotta look at that. How is this affecting the families? Our future? Because two hundred people here is a lot. It's a big section. What [the government] gonna do for them girls, not just the ones that they bury, the ones that still living with it for however long. What else is going to happen to their bodies? Can they get pregnant?

I offer Bee's comments at length because they comprehensively trace the intimacies among anxieties around the vaccine, reproduction, and futurity and the close relationship between the country's future, the former government's agreed-on ineffectiveness, and the pervasive effects of globalization in Barbados—from the penetration of American television and fashion to the government's welcome embrace of an influx of pharmaceutical and multinational companies motivated by profit. Linking the vaccine and its side effects to the potential death of Barbadian children, Bee insists we consider not only her daughter's future but the country's futurity should the government continue promoting the vaccine. Her wariness that those promoting the vaccine would be unwilling and unable to assist her family should her daughter have a negative response to the vaccine was similarly echoed above by Naitry, who lamented, "It is *my* daughter who would have to live with the consequences."

Randall, a young father mentioned in chapter 1, expressed similar frustrations about the promotion of the vaccine in "small" Barbados, which he felt was commonly in a position of inferiority, frequently subject to the force and influence of the United States and powerful multinational companies. For Randall, the Barbadian government was merely a "puppet"—complicit with economic motives of large companies and countries, often at the expense of citizens' well-being:

By me saying that I am not going to protect, as they call it "protect" my child and the children of this country with the HPV vaccine that they are providing, I am effectively saying to them that I have an issue with possibly maiming or killing my child. We are small, we are insignificant, we have little power, we have little to offer, so that's why we would almost always find ourselves in situations like this. We've been conditioned to believe or to accept that it *has* to be done. It's almost being forced down our throat. It's like [the government] is saying, "You must have it, otherwise you can't go to school," or the Big Pharma companies saying, "You must have it, otherwise this or that."

Randall's concerns about the vaccine's effect on his child's life are tied to those around the capitalistic motivations of the pharmaceutical company promoting the vaccine and the sense of force he felt the government projected and has historically used to control, persuade, and condition its citizens to accept biopolitical measures in the name of health and protection.

In response to my curiosity about nurses' experiences interacting with these parents and responding to concerns over the financial motives of the pharmaceutical company and the potential long-term effects of the vaccine on Barbadian youth and young women's fertility, Nurse Parker shared with me:

> Well, some were wary about the side effects they heard about, about children being paralyzed, you know, what they read online. And there were some well-known people in Barbados who made comments about us not wanting the vaccine to affect our children in later life and we don't know what effects this vaccine will have ten years down the road. Is it really protecting against cancer? What about infertility? a good few were asking. Are the drug companies just making money? I try to tell them, "Listen, this vaccine is not new. This vaccine is being given all around the world. We are not the first, we are not the test subjects, we are probably one of the last ones who are now getting it, okay. And it's a very expensive vaccine that our government is covering. There is nothing that is available in this world that someone isn't making a profit from, okay?" So I try to show them that sense. Even natural remedies, you will read about online, people make money off those too. And another question they ask too is, "Would you give it to your child?" and well I have told parents, that listen, I took it myself. There is not a vaccine in here that I administer that I haven't actually had myself.

Rather than clarifying statistics on the vaccine's efficacy or speaking directly to parents' concerns about their children's futurity, Nurse Parker's response tries to normalize the financial motives of the pharmaceutical company promoting the vaccine in an inescapably capitalist world. It is well-intentioned but ultimately dismissive responses like these to which parents noted feeling that their concerns were overlooked by medical professionals, creating further discomfort and unease. Yet the significance of the relationship between these parents' concerns about the vaccine's association with reproduction and futurity and histories of racialized subjectivity, reproductive violence, and capitalism under slavery cannot be overstated. Tracing specific histories and itineraries of risk and suspicion in the British Caribbean, during slavery and after emancipation, I argued in chapter 2 for a recognition of suspicion as an affective intensity that is contemporarily experienced by Afro-Barbadian citizens in a political economy inextricably linked to capitalist accumulation and extraction on behalf of the colonial and the postcolonial state. In this economy, suspicion and biopolitical mediation of and on the Black woman's reproductive body are palimpsests, exceeding linear time and national borders.

In her book of poetry, *Patient*, Bettina Judd interweaves her personal medical history with the historical evidence of scientific racism and medical experiments on Black women during the nineteenth-century United States, to meditate on the persistent acuity of these injustices on Black women's experiences with the health care system today.[11] Like the suspicion experienced by the Afro-Caribbean parents I interviewed, the mistrust, skepticism, fear, and anger Judd poetically details are residues and affects that, though deeply resonant for many Black women, remain overwhelmingly overlooked or disbelieved in contemporary medical contexts. Analogizing the disregard for the psychic toll of these sordid histories on Black women's experiences with health to the denial of Black people's everyday experience of racism, Judd states, "It's like when a black person says, 'That's racist' to a white person and they refuse to believe. Maybe it is better to say, 'This moment is steeped in a racist history. This racist history is indelibly imprinted on my memory. You do not want to remember, so you wish to erase mine.'[12] Saidiya Hartman reiterates these connections, describing how flesh and reproduction, both "produced by the violence of racial slavery," remain central to contemporary deliberations about Black women's material relations in the afterlife of slavery and in the context of global capitalism.[13] Indeed, when we read these parents' embodied narratives of suspicion, gut feelings, and bad senses about the vaccine, its forceful promotion, and the perceived threat it poses to reproduction and futurity, we see a refraction of the colonial suspicions, biopolitical interventions, and modes of violence under slavery and in the postslavery period. We can largely discern this from these parents even in the absence of overt mentions of slavery. Instead, connecting their concerns about the vaccine and its effects on reproductive futurity to anxieties around the country's small size, the state's increasing apathy, and involvement in global assemblages, parents trace a narrative that connects the long history of racialized exploitation and biopower in the Caribbean with contemporary state and biomedical attempts to protect reproduction, via vaccination, through the skin and flesh.

The skin, as Sara Ahmed and Jackie Stacey note, is "that fleshy interface between bodies and worlds" that materializes in multiple forms, opening our bodies to outer feeling, touch, force, beautification, desire, and increasingly medical intervention.[14] It is also that object produced through what Frantz Fanon calls epidermalization, that, according to Paul Gilroy, describes the "historically specific system for making bodies meaningful by endowing them with qualities of 'color.'"[15] Skin and flesh have been made to signal race, and through this process, the Black body has been denied its humanity. Puncturing the skin and flesh, vaccines enter our bodies with the forceful jab of a needle. There is pain, there is swelling, there is redness. Most of us know someone who fears or avoids needles for this very reason. Yet the Afro-Barbadian parents with whom I spoke drew on this language of pain and force to refer not to the insertion of the needle into the skin but to the forceful strength and intensity with which they sensed the Ministry of Health, its doctors, and nurses were using to "shove it down their throats," through their flesh, and into their sensing, mindful bodies.

Emphasizing the importance of flesh for theorizing the cultural continuation of slavery, Black transatlantic scholars reiterate that this Black flesh was marked, beaten, scored, and branded as a saleable commodity and object to be traded, bought, and sold.[16] A tabula rasa on which slavery inscribes itself, flesh, Spillers is clear to note, is antecedent to the body. In her influential essay, "Mama's Baby, Papa's Maybe: An American Grammar Book," she argues, "before the 'body' there is 'flesh'"—making a distinction between the Black female body and its flesh, which was demarcated and objectified in an attempt for Blackness to be unmade into a racialized commodity.[17] It is "these undecipherable markings on the captive body," this "hieroglyphics of the flesh," Spillers says, that gave rise to a grammar that continues to demonize and make fungible Black women and men today.[18] Thus for Spillers, flesh can and ought to be thought of as the "primary narrative" of embodiment, as that which emphasizes Black subjectivity as humanity.[19] Here, flesh is understood, as it is by Chicana feminists Cherríe Moraga and Gloria Anzaldúa, as critical to a necessary political theory of survival for women and people of color. Through the flesh, blood, and as I argue the gut, Afro-Barbadian parents make sense of the vaccine; the historical, affective memories of slavery; and the racialized capitalist logics that they perceive to inhere in the HPV vaccine and its promotion. Understanding these suspicions as and in the erotic, as affective, as sensible, and as a form of sensing complicates biomedical narratives around suspicion and hesitancy as irrational refusals of protection.

Sensing force in the vaccine's promotion, unsettled by, re-membering, and feeling histories and residues of suspicious affects in and through the body—the mind, the gut, the skin, the flesh—Afro-Barbadian parents with whom I spoke collectively narrated a sensibility of suspicion that was at once a sensibility about protection. For these parents, suspicion worked to shield their children from all that was unknown about the vaccine, including its side effects, the motivations behind its production, and the state's priorities in promoting it to the Barbadian public. Cognizant of the implications of these fraught understandings of protection for the health of the young men and women whose parents refused vaccination, the doctors and nurses I interviewed relayed their efforts to encourage parents to "come to their senses" by trusting the medical sensibility of vaccination as protection. Yet simply reiterating claims to medical certainty without seriously addressing (and at times erasing) parents' most salient concerns seemed only to fuel parents' suspicions and affirm the desire to protect their children. In the chapter's final parts, I closely explore this notion of protection as expressed to me by Afro-Barbadian parents via suspicion.

Suspicion and/as Protection

Harriet is a thirty-four-year-old Afro-Barbadian engineer and mother of four children. She developed genital warts from HPV while pregnant with her first daughter. Because of the size of the warts on her vaginal walls, Harriet's doctors recommended she have a caesarean section delivery to reduce complications and to mitigate the possibility of warts being passed on to her daughter during birth. Unable to make it to the hospital in time for a caesarean, Harriet had a vaginal birth, and a few months later, her daughter began developing a large wart in her mouth. Recalling the discovery of her daughter's wart twelve years ago and her recent education about the HPV vaccine via TV advertisements, Harriet shared,

> My poor child, she was only one year old and had this big growth in her mouth. I knew right away it was the same HPV. So she was admitted to the ear, nose and throat specialist at the hospital and she had a surgery to remove this growth.... The doctors never really told me much, but they did tell me it was a small possibility when I delivered her vaginally that she could contract it. So then when I heard of the vaccine on TV a couple years ago, I saw they said they were giving it to girls before they reached a sexual age, around eleven years, and I was confused. I knew that my daughter was exposed from birth. So I began reading up on the vaccine online and the majority of things I was finding were people talking about the negative consequences and complications of receiving it so I thought this was strange and thought, why not take the vaccine off the market right now if there are all these side effects? Why not check on it some more? Because these are girls!

When I asked Harriet to elaborate on her concern about the safety of the vaccine for girls in particular, she emphasized the difference with which "us women are made to deal with things" compared to boys and men, and how important it was to protect young girls because "they will carry our children." "It's just different," she said, and the potential effects of the vaccine on her daughter's reproductive abilities, especially after having already contracted HPV from her, were too great a risk:

I'm protecting all my children now, not just my oldest daughter, from getting this shot that hasn't been researched enough. I have asked questions to other parents who have been exposed to HPV, I have done Google searches, and I'm not just going with anything I see online, I go back to original sources and dig deep to see where the information is coming from. I eventually told my daughter's friends' parents that I had decided no and encouraged them to do further research. Basically, what it comes down to is that I feel like my daughter was exposed to it already and I don't want to put her in more harm, but also, you know, I had something to do with her getting HPV initially and so now I have a choice to protect her from other harm and I don't want her to have this vaccine that needs more research.

Like many Afro-Barbadian mothers mentioned in chapter 3, Harriet's words reveal long-standing gendered ideologies around women and societal expectations regarding women's reproduction such that protection of women in particular ought to be prioritized for these purposes. Contextualizing her decision to refuse the vaccine in terms of the guilt she felt about transmitting HPV to her daughter and her fear of further harm in the form of a new vaccination, Harriet offers an understanding of protection achieved through a refusal of the vaccine, an ethical choice that emerged from suspicions and uncertainties about the vaccine's safety and her desires to protect her child's reproductive system.

Having had a similar prior experience with HPV, Simone refused the vaccine for her daughter because her discomfort around government and industry economic alliances and the increasing power pharmaceutical companies seemed to have over the public's health. In her late teens, Simone tested positive for abnormal cervical cells during a routine Pap smear and underwent cryotherapy to destroy her precancerous cells. Since then, she has received Pap smears regularly and described herself as a staunch advocate for this test as the best chance for detecting cervical cancer. In this context, she framed her suspicion and subsequent refusal of the HPV vaccine and its forceful imposition on the Barbadian public and young women in particular:

My resentment comes in part from, you know, the promotion. . . . It's like a Macy's launch of a new product, and [it] was being pushed so hard. When I looked at the some of the ads on TV, the tone of it was, "a responsible parent vaccinates for this," as opposed to, "a responsible parent encourages their child to get Pap smears." Immediately, all I thought was, why didn't they ever push Pap smears in that way? Why didn't they ever push, you know, women sitting and talking to their daughter? Why didn't they push that, you know? Governments and pharmaceutical companies have all this money and different agendas.... The thing is that I cannot actually blame the industry because I think what it plays on is people's general unknowingness and worry . . . and women specifically are a demographic that spend money on medication and on health care, so it's a good demographic to invest in. But [the industry has] problematized something that need not be a problem. Yes, cervical cancer is a concern. But . . . I know that the process between catching cells and being diagnosed with cervical cancer is one that's not inevitable.... If you are doing your Pap and catching abnormal cells . . . they say it is one of the best cancers to have, right? . . . Cervical cancer takes a long time to develop. So you have a long window during which you can spot an abnormal cell, you can act on the presence of an abnormal cell rather than teaching your daughter that a vaccine will protect her. Teach her and protect her in that way. That is unless she has a very aggressive form, okay, unless hers is extremely aggressive, and in which case I don't know that a vaccine would help you anyway.

Simone asks critical questions of the Barbadian government and its investment in fervently promoting this pharmaceutical product without equal regard, past or present, for the promotion of Pap smears, which remain medically the best chance to detect most cervical cancers. Simultaneously suspicious and clairvoyant about the state, medical, and pharmaceutical conceptions of protection through vaccination, Simone offers an alternate vision of protection, one that is partly based on her lived experiences with precancerous cells and the information she has learned about the power and importance of Pap smears.[20] In this framing, protection is achieved through transmitting this embodied knowledge to her daughter, informing her about her sexual health risks, and presenting an understanding of responsible health care decision making in the form of Pap smears. Simone is not unique in having personal experiences with precancerous cells, and expressing an understanding of protection that in part stems from an education about a woman's body and sexual health risks.

Tricia is a forty-year-old artist and mother of two who was also exposed to high-risk strains of HPV in her teens, which were detected early through a Pap smear. "For me," she notes, "there is nothing to stop you from being healthy, from having children afterward and living a long life once you detect it early through Paps." Tricia attributes much of her decision to refuse the vaccine for her daughter to her firsthand experiences with HPV. She explained, "It's not that I want her to go through that, I mean no parent ever does. But my parents didn't talk to me about that [HPV] . . . and I can easily say, 'Hey, mummy had this, I've dealt with this, and you're not invincible. . . . This can all happen to us, I've been there and I don't want to scare you but it's possible that it could happen to you, too.'" Though both Tricia's children received routine immunizations as infants, she felt the HPV vaccine was problematic because she believed that educating her daughter about HPV and instructing her on the value of Pap smears were important lessons to impart about protection—lessons she also felt should be prioritized over a choice to receive a vaccine. "An education, not a vaccine, is what you owe to your children. You have to be confident in your ability as a parent to know that your job is to make your children independent and knowledgeable to protect themselves, and that's probably one of the biggest things for me with this vaccine that makes me concerned. Because this thing [cervical cancer] is so preventable."

It was initially surprising to me that 20 percent of the Barbadian mothers I interviewed about the HPV vaccine had their own previous nerve-wracking experiences with HPV yet ultimately refused the vaccine for their children. I took for granted the belief these mothers shared about their own power in protecting their daughters by educating them about sex and sexual health and relaying their missteps and stories about HPV in their lives so that their daughters might lead less vulnerable lives. A closer engagement with these parents' words reveals that their understandings of protection are inextricably and intimately connected to past lived (and painful) experiences with HPV and a subsequent emergent ethics of responsibility to shield their daughters from unknown side effects while educating them about their bodies and their sexual health as the foremost form of defense and protection.

We might align Simone's, Tricia's, and Harriet's embodied knowledges and their conceptions of protection through a transmission of this lived experience with claims of other Afro-Barbadian parents like Janine and Bee, whose suspicions toward the vaccine emphasize related embodied senses of knowledge around futurity and reproduction. For Janine and Bee, embodied and enfleshed senses of memory around the racialized and reproductive violence of capitalism and slavery attach suspicions to biocapitalistic products like the HPV vaccine introduced by the postcolonial state. Guided by embodied sensibilities, for these parents protection looks to and centers their children's futures in light of these critical pasts. Further echoing parents like Randall, Denise, and Darcy, who expressed discomfort with the forceful promotion of the vaccine and questioned their government's interests beyond seeking to protect citizens, Simone and Tricia, if implicitly, suggest a protection formulated in response and in relation to the suspicious medicopharmaceutical state and its biopolitical priorities.

Pat, a thirty-five-year-old mother of two girls, most clearly articulated this relationship between Afro-Barbadian parents, the government, and the formation of protection when she explained her reasoning behind refusing the vaccine for her twelve-year-old daughter:

> In my son's school, things like gastroenteritis would spread rampant because a lot of public schools do not have toilet paper, they don't have soap, you understand me? You have to give your child sanitizer, send them with sanitizer, soap, I give her wipes. . . . That's how they do it here. So when you get alarmed when gastro starts and spreads rampant . . . jeez, like, it's so backward. The private schools might be a bit different because you know, you got parents who pay. But not with our government and our government schools. I remember too when my daughter was in preschool there was a primary school located on the same property. Eventually the primary school moved and they took the security with them. So the children remaining who are special needs kids and the little ones (a maximum of three years old) were left with no security and the government did not see the need to address it. . . . How dare you? The government would say, "Oh we can't afford to send a security guard to protect the children" when people of all walks of life was using the abandoned [primary school] building to live in and endangering the children. I am not no anti-vaxxer by any means. But, with the Gardasil, I seen those stories online, and I don't want her to be the guinea pig. . . . And even if that Gardasil protected against all strains of HPV then it would maybe make me think twice, but telling me well she can't get these two kinds but she could get the other five or whatever it is, on top of everything else with [this government], makes me question this next push for protection.

Identifying several cases where the government failed to provide protection for her children's health and safety, Pat calls attention to the unevenness of the state's biopolitics, which, for her, cast significant doubt on its priorities when it comes to truly protecting citizens. In light of a lack of basic sanitary measures and security in schools, she is forced to question the state's seemingly limited medicopharmaceutical conception of protection as achieved through a biomedical drug. By questioning this logic, Pat subsequently casts doubt on the intensity of the HPV vaccination program, the use of her daughter as a guinea pig, and the scientific efficacy of the vaccine in preventing cervical cancer—concerns shared and sensed by parents like Denise, David, Bee, and Naitry. For Pat, as for most of these parents, refusal emerges from a multiplicity of suspicions and skepticisms around the government's view of protection and commitment to its citizens. Protection, as clearly referred to here by Pat, Tricia, and

Simone, is a thoughtful ethics, formulated from a dutiful relationship to the past and the future, and through the complex interactions between postcolonial citizens and parents like themselves, and the Barbadian state, the economy, and its enmeshment in biopolitical pharmaceutical assemblages. In the words of Audre Lorde, such epistemologies, ethics of protection, and survivability are achieved through a "disciplined" and sincere attention and commitment to one's deepest feelings and sensibilities, which are "sanctuaries and spawning grounds for the most radical and daring of ideas," and thus should not be thought of as "idle fantasy."[21] These epistemologies further circulate in and foreground the exploitative transnational economics and politics that constitute and are constituted by the HPV vaccine.

Suspicion around the HPV vaccine thus operates as an affective sensibility to instill in Afro-Barbadian parents particular ethical imperatives and epistemologies of protection—narratives and knowledges that rub up against those espoused by the government and the pharmaceutical industry as sensible. The government and Big Pharma are invested in the vaccine's promotion and acceptance and believe that protection is achieved through the rational choice to vaccinate one's child. Rather than ambivalence toward vaccination reflecting an "irrational" form of resistance, parents' suspicion is an embodied, corporeal affect that calls into question the protection offered by the vaccine and its effects on women's reproduction and futurity in ways that disconnect these citizens from the ideas, people, and objects deemed suspicious and untrustworthy. As parents detail, suspicion is protective not just from the vaccine and its unknown side effects but against Big Pharma, the perceived financial motivations of government–industry partnerships, and the state's overarching interests in the health care of its citizens. In this way, suspicion as protection is an ethics that complexly confronts the state's biopolitics and priorities to ethically protect and educate Barbadians. And yet, suspicion is fraught.

Although most HPV infections are asymptomatic and clear without treatment, persistent infection with high-risk strains of HPV can develop into precancerous lesions, cervical cancer, head and neck cancers, and genital cancers. The Caribbean is currently among the top four highest subregions in the world with respect to the incidence of cervical cancer and has the highest burden of HPV in the Americas. In a context where care for and about cervical cancer is urgent, suspicion's potential to engender refusal of the HPV vaccine inevitably threatens attempts to save lives. Continued low HPV vaccine uptake rates can have grave health repercussions for the young women and men whose parents are seeking to protect them via suspicion and refusal of the vaccine. Indeed, suspicion is impossibly imperfect, and although it might offer protection in multiple senses, it might also engender the refusal of life-saving interventions, resulting in disease or death.

Still it is true that danger lies in pathologizing Afro-Barbadian parents' suspicion and hesitancy toward the HPV vaccine as something to be summarily overlooked and eradicated, as it does in viewing vaccination as the sole means of sensibility. Invoking affective memories of the past, parents' "hesitancy" asks of the motivations behind the biomedical offerings of care presented via the HPV vaccine and, in so doing, reveals care's inequalities and political stakes by mapping how health care work, biomedical authority, state priorities, assemblages, and noninnocent histories of colonial medical injustice often unwittingly intertwine. Perhaps, as Michelle Murphy encourages, we ought to resist the urge to wholly conflate understandings of care and protection with positive affects.[22] Indeed, like the "grammar" that has historically overdetermined Black women as hypersexual, deviant, and in need of care and salvation, the dominant "grammar" of vaccine hesitancy overwhelmingly, inadvertently, and paternalistically naturalizes protection and care via vaccination as uncomplicatedly benevolent.[23]

As Hiʻilei Hobart and Tamara Kneese remind us, we might think instead of radical care as an omnipresent obligation, built on a set of ethical, political, and collective strategies toward an otherwise.[24] Black feminist theory's longstanding investment in embodiment as a means through which Black women practice this ethics of radical care and survival is testament to the struggle and necessity of resisting colonial and scientific claims to objectivity and rationality and insisting on, as Jennifer Nash writes, the deeply "sensual, spiritual, creative, and corporeal ways of knowing."[25] Through suspicion, an affective and corporeal form of protection, the Afro-Barbadian parents quoted herein demonstrate what it means to instrumentalize this collective capacity for caring otherwise, beyond those modeled to us in persistent colonial capitalisms. A willingness to interrogate the dominant scripts around care and protection recognizes suspicion's fallible nature and opens up the space to rewire our approach to the sensibility of suspicion as something that ought to be overcome by virtue of it being fraught. Such a move might instead usher in a sense of reflection on suspicion's gestures toward experiential knowledge and less injurious forms of health care promotion. Chapter 5 continues to explore suspicion's generativity amid its shortcomings and investigates its relationship to the biomedical certainty espoused by Barbadian medical practitioners. Illustrating the simultaneously productive and fallible nature of suspicion and certainty, I argue for the generative insights they collectively offer public health practitioners and scholars seeking to understand the racialized, gendered, historical, and affective politics of care and its presumed impediments.

FIVE

Suspicion and Certainty

In my interviews with Barbadian medical professionals and parents, both spoke passionately about the plethora of information about the HPV vaccine that circulated online, including pictures, blog posts, and videos that were posted to Facebook and a series of websites created by parents internationally to urge others to reconsider the vaccine and lobby their respective governments to suspend its promotion.[1] For doctors and nurses these sites were dangerous forms of clickbait filled with antivaccination rhetoric and propaganda, whereas the parents I interviewed collectively viewed these forums as powerful spaces in which they could see reflected their embodied sensibilities of suspicion around the HPV vaccine, the intensity with which they felt it was forced on them, and what they perceived to be the government's questionable motivations behind its promotion.

One of the stories shared widely across these online forums and mentioned to me by several mothers and nurses was that of a twelve-year-old girl named Briar from New Zealand, who received her first dose of the HPV vaccine in May 2014. According to her mother's post on the nonprofit website Gardasil Awareness NZ, a few months after her first shot, Briar experienced severe and sustained symptoms of headaches, dizziness, chest pain, fatigue, and anxiety, leading a team of doctors to diagnose her with chronic fatigue syndrome, fibromyalgia, and complex regional pain syndrome, which they did not directly associate with the HPV vaccine.[2] In a video, a young Briar wails on her bed, unable to stand, and pleads with her mother to let her remain lying down. "This was a very hard video to post, my twelve-year-old daughter was fine before her vaccine, now this is her life.... I'm showing this because I want people to know what damage this vaccine can and does cause. Please research before deciding. *I didn't....*" her mother passionately warns. So compelling were such unverifiable posts for parents like thirty-nine-year-old Bee that watching Briar in pain was research enough to decide that she would refuse the vaccine for her daughter:

NICOLE: Did you do more research online since you first heard about the HPV vaccine and saw Briar's video?

BEE: No ... umm ... well, actually the first thing I read online said that one or two people died and that, then, is therefore a possibility and so to me it is not worth it. And then I saw this video of Briar. So I don't have to ask anybody else. I made a decision right then. What's the point? I could go talk to whoever and whoever people who got it and nothing happened them, good for them. But even if you say it's only 3 percent of these people that something happened to after taking the vaccine, for those 3 percent it is their life 100 percent, and if you're my only daughter and you are one of the 3 percent, my whole world collapse[s]. The 97 percent ain't got nothing to do with me. If she could be dead and she's mine, then no. They cannot be risking or sacrificing these few (if you call it a few), to protect some. Because that little girl that I saw on Facebook from New Zealand, who some days she cannot get up off her bed after this vaccine ... that hurts.

NICOLE: So it's the perceived side effects that you have witnessed online in such videos that make the vaccine just not worth the risk?

BEE: Look. She is crippled and she cannot do anything much. Her mother is not going to be able to take a job because she is going to be home with her ... and you not going to know how it will be down the line, this is only her initial reaction. I think she got [the HPV vaccine] two years ago and it was a series of three shots and she got all three, so she has been living like this for a year now.

While Briar's mother suggests that the HPV vaccine is related to the onset of the extensive list of conditions her daughter experienced, neither Merck nor the CDC has listed any information to scientifically correlate the Gardasil quadrivalent vaccine to fibromyalgia, chronic fatigue syndrome, complex pain syndrome, or any such symptoms/side effects.[3] Still, as Bee shares, the mere sight of Briar in pain was powerful enough to confirm her suspicions, guiding her to decline the vaccine. Though she refused the protection the vaccine promised her daughter, Bee nonetheless believes her decision to be protective because it safeguards her daughter from the pain and suffering she witnessed in the video.

Clare, another Afro-Barbadian mother, shared a similar experience in response to this same video. Clare expressed feeling uneasy about the way Barbadian nurses were pushing the vaccine on parents. When I asked if she did any research to learn more about the HPV vaccine, she admitted to merely browsing the internet, where she stumbled upon Briar's story:

> I did research it online and then I looked up the side effects of it and then I saw this video from the UK or New Zealand I think. Yeah, and I saw a mother that had given her daughter the vaccination and the excruciating pain that little girl was going through just to do simple things. I mean, she couldn't even move her legs. The action of actually trying to get her to move her legs was so painful that she was crying and screaming for her mother to stop. That for me is cementing the decision that I don't want it for her ... for my daughter. Because I don't want to take that chance. And I did some more research on it too apart from that video, I read and watched more videos on it, and every day on Facebook I am seeing some child or the other died. ... I am against it.

Sharing her concerns about videos like Briar's and the internet more generally, immunization Nurse Alleyne noted with frustration:

> In Barbados especially, people tend to look to what goes on in the wider world, right ... so because Australia had reported they had over one thousand cases of various adverse reactions, [Barbadians] took that to heart and that was one of the reasons why the intake here was not as good as it should be.
>
> NICOLE: Was this something parents expressed seeing or reading about on Facebook?
>
> NURSE ALLEYNE: Facebook and Google. They went on the internet, they read, and the internet was gospel. Nothing we said could change it because, "Uh uh this and that and the internet said this, and, no." And I kept telling people, well you don't use Wikipedia as any source of reference when you're studying, right? So ... And you found parents with limited education, sorry to say, they just catch excerpts from wherever, from the periphery or whatever, and they don't even understand what they see but they come up with this horror story and then at one time, there was this highlight about this teenager in Australia who went into anaphylactic shock and was so sick, and

who had mental challenges and so on. And a lot of people focused on that. That example came up over and over and as some parents said, there's nothing we could say or do to convince them otherwise. Not right now or later.

Reminding us of the transnational influence of foreign states, industries, and businesses in Barbados and of the simultaneous interest many Barbadians have in transnational affairs outside the Barbadian state, Nurse Alleyne underscores the affective intensity of online videos and claims made by parents in places like Australia and points to the dangers they might pose to Barbadians at risk for HPV. Although she appears to believe these forums have more resonance for those with "limited education," my discussions with primarily middle-class Afro-Barbadian parents highlight that keeping track of and paying attention to what happens outside Barbados is key for many to monitor their own suspicions about their government, its abuse of authority, its commitment to citizens' rights, and its complicity in for-profit global assemblages.

Many Afro-Barbadians who browsed the internet for information on the HPV vaccine encountered what they perceived to be truthful and reliable communities of parents around the world asking questions, sharing links to other groups, and expressing a commitment to protect their children from the vaccine and the governments, industries, and professionals promoting it. Many described the discussion boards as sought-after spaces where they could share, explore, and validate their gut feelings and suspicions about the vaccine—sensibilities they wanted to keep private from friends and doctors for fear of being ridiculed. This form of transnational community building and exploration—forged by suspicion and facilitated through the internet—was crucial in 2016 in a place like Barbados, whose economy was still recovering from the 2008 global financial crisis, whose government was concurrently proposing invasive biometric screening for all those entering and leaving the country, and whose citizens' skepticism around the foreign and economic influence on the state was widespread. As with the HPV vaccination program, citizens' response to the proposed biometric screening program was met with an analysis of international and transnational politics in an attempt to justify what the government should and should not be doing with its own citizens. As one father, Randall, claimed about his online research about the HPV vaccine, it was largely by looking outside the nation-state and to transnational communities of parents from more developed, more powerful, and internationally recognized places like Australia, New Zealand, and the United Kingdom that parents like himself felt affirmed in their suspicions and confident to question the Barbadian state and its networks of medicopharmaceutical assemblages via suspicion or refusal of the vaccine.

With little more uniting parents like Bee and Randall to Briar's mother besides their young children, the HPV vaccine, and the affects of suspicion it engenders, doctors and nurses are right to point to the affectively charged and disconcerting nature of home videos like Briar's and associated HPV vaccine social media groups for the negative influence they can have on HPV vaccine compliance. At the same time, social media groups and videos ought not—by virtue of their existence—be considered "fake," as they are often proclaimed to be by many Barbadian medical professionals.

This chapter seeks to problematize this linkage between HPV vaccination hesitancy, fake news, and antivaccination/antiscience rhetoric to situate and investigate the projections of biomedical certainty emerging through this discursive process. Although this book's focus so far has been to examine suspicion as simultaneously generative and fraught, much remains to be interrogated around the discourses of certainty espoused by medical professionals, what they elide and obscure, and their relationship with discourses of suspicion. Detailing the comments made by medical professionals and parents about certainty and suspicion, I explore the precarious binary constructed between the two. In this untenable binary, we lose sight of the shortcomings of suspicion and certainty and the generativity they collectively offer transnational scholars of affect and public health practitioners working in an increasingly digital, neoliberal, fake news, and post-truth era.[4] Complementing the transnational and women of color feminist study of affect I have theorized in this book to include feminist sociologist Arlie Hochschild's theorizations of "feeling rules," I gesture toward the multiple subjectivities and ethics of care that derive from certainty and suspicion and offer an understanding of them as relational rather than oppositional.[5] Situating parents' ideologies of suspicion, protection, and claims to self-determination in the context of Caribbean feminist and Afro-diasporic activism and advocacy around racialized communities' health from the 1970s to 1990s, I consider the transformative potential biomedical certainty and suspicion promise for improved public health promotion of HPV and its related diseases in Barbados.

Suspicion and Fake News Online

In May 2019, the CDC reported the greatest number of cases in measles in the United States in a single year in nearly three decades as a result of declining rates of vaccination.[6] Alongside such disconcerting trends and resulting public health efforts to increase vaccine compliance by cautioning against the dangers of vaccine refusal has been a related shift in the discourse surrounding hesitancy.

Defined in 2011 by the WHO as the temporary delay or complete refusal of vaccines in the context of available immunization services, vaccine hesitancy is increasingly framed by medical journalists, commentators, and public health professionals as a growing trend of mistrust, misinformation, and public ignorance in and about vaccines that emerges online.[7] In North American and European contexts in particular, claims to public ignorance often headline discussions of vaccine hesitancy across medical news forums and newspaper editorials, driving a narrative that uncritically conflates hesitancy with refusal and frames these phenomena as collective consequences of fearful, misguided, science-skeptic citizens who traffic in the dangerous online world of fake news. Across such accounts, public ignorance is widely believed to be perpetuated by antivaccination propaganda, specifically the notorious 1998 Wakefield *Lancet* study and its accompanying scandal, which fraudulently showed links between autism and the MMR vaccine. Though this study, the doctor, and the science behind it have been widely discredited, Wakefield et al.'s claims laid the foundation for the formation of contemporary antivaccine groups and a broader movement across North America and the United Kingdom.[8] As Maya Goldenberg describes, such groups, made up of "self-serving researchers and celebrity spokespeople, mobilized parent groups desperate to lay blame for their children's autism, and a sensationalist media," effectively and problematically "fa[n] the flames of public mistrust of the scientific consensus."[9] Indeed, as groups of antivaxxers and imagery of primarily white, educated, upper-middle-class citizens with "alternative lifestyles" who refuse vaccines for fears of disability increasingly saturate contemporary online channels and popular science texts, so does the wider public (health) imaginary about vaccine hesitancy progressively become associated with fake news and online propaganda.[10] "While measles may be the disease," executive director of UNICEF Henrietta Fore illustratively notes, "the real infection is misinformation," adding to a chorus of voices calling for an antidote to the medicopolitical antivaxxer virus that is vaccine hesitancy.[11]

When I first began writing this book in the wake of the 2016 US presidential election, concerns were just beginning to swarm the media around the influence of fake news on the election and its increasing capacity to distort a series of social and political incidents globally.[12] More worrisome than rumor or incorrect (potentially accidental) sources of misinformation, fake news is distinguishable for its "intentionally and verifiably false" disinformation, which often follows the conventions of reputable journalism to create the impression of validity.[13] Amid the then-widespread international public hysteria around online fake news articles, cautioning parents against turning to social media and the internet for verifiable information about the HPV vaccine became central to the Barbadian Ministry of Health's messaging. "Ignore Internet" states a renowned local gynecologist at the Queen Elizabeth Hospital in a piece written for the *Nation News*, urging parents to follow the advice of medical professionals to vaccinate their daughters and warning against the dangers of online forums. In my interviews, doctors and nurses reiterated this concern around the growing popularity of social media as a source of medical (dis)information. Alongside international public health efforts to mitigate the influence of growing antivaccination online forums, Barbadian health professionals decried these groups and the internet writ large, believing them to be directly associated with fake news and parents' feelings of suspicion and hesitancy toward the HPV vaccine.

Through this seemingly benign discursive process of linking vaccine hesitancy with antivaccination rhetoric and fake news, several entwined material and ideological moves are accomplished. First, the nuanced beliefs, histories, and emotions of parents who express hesitancy in different regions in relation to particular vaccines are obscured. In the Barbadian context, this move elides the voices of the predominantly Afro-Barbadians with whom this book is concerned—for whom suspicion attaches to the HPV vaccine, its pharmaceutical manufacturers and state administrators, the uncharacteristic way it was introduced and promoted across the island, colonial tropes of Black women's hypersexuality, and related histories of biomedical injustice and experimentation on Black women from the period of slavery. By overlooking these complex politics, affects, and histories, I argue, vaccine hesitancy becomes effectively and dangerously conflated with antivaccine sentiment–*cum*-disinformation and fake news. Through this process, vaccination and its benefits are heralded as authoritative modes of absolute truth and certainty—the antithesis of suspicion, which ought to be eliminated rather than examined for the insights it might offer public health practitioners and scholars.

While vaccine hesitancy might exist alongside antivaccine sentiment for some people, the two ought not be conflated. As this book has detailed, for instance, suspicion is less an active attempt to resist the HPV vaccine and more an embodied feeling/affect that attaches to technologies like the vaccine, its promotion, and its complex neoliberal, postcolonial, gendered, and racialized politics. While for many of the Afro-Barbadian parents with whom I spoke suspicion did engender refusal of the vaccine, it simultaneously asked questions (and fostered its own understandings) of care and protection, histories of injurious biopolitics under slavery's system of racialized and gendered capitalism, and the Barbadian state's accountability to its citizens amid its enmeshment in global state–industry assemblages. By subsuming parents' suspicion in the rubric of fake news, medical professionals effectively obscure these realities and possibilities.

For instance, consider Nurse Jane, who felt strongly that the Ministry of Health's efforts to increase vaccination coverage and protect citizens were being sidelined by parents' blind and widespread reliance on the internet and the ease of access to fake news therein:

> To some extent parents aren't really sitting and thinking about this, you know. Some of them are making decisions without checking things, just blindly saying no. You know? Instead of reading up. You know how it is with the internet now. They go on different sites and see that this thing is killing people and this [person] died from this and all sorts of things they hearing. Some of them were too much you know. One parent told me that they saw on the net that after taking the HPV vaccine this child had some sort of really horrible reaction. So you know how that kind of fake news spreads and makes people even more skeptical to take things that will protect them.

These comments suggest that any negative thoughts and press around the HPV vaccine contained online are fake news and that Barbadian parents are largely undiscerning online consumers for whom fake news has dangerous repercussions. In many cases, the line between misinformation about the HPV vaccine and antiscience/antivaccine disinformation can often be quite blurred. For instance, although many of the nonprofit websites linked to social media groups on the HPV vaccine were created by parents whose aim was to share their children's painful experiences after receiving the vaccine, some of these sites contained links that redirect users to antivaccine sites rife with antiscience claims and fake news stories disguised in pseudoscientific discourse. It is deciphering the subtleties between fake news and accurate journalism or peer-reviewed research and developing a sense of internet literacy about which some health care professionals were understandably wary. Many expressed concern for parents like Bee, who felt so tenaciously convinced in the harm the vaccine could instill after viewing only one parent's video that she did not feel the need to consult with any medical practitioners.

Such professionals' concerns about misinformation and fake news were met with further suspicions from many parents who were convinced that different motivations lay behind their purported apprehensions. Reflecting on medical professionals' warnings against the internet as a source of reliable information about the HPV vaccine, David commented on the threat his internet research and occasional browsing of online discussion boards seemed to pose to his doctor's sense of authority:

DAVID: They think we dumb! Listen, I am not a medical expert but I feel that sometimes doctors feel that they have you at an advantage, and if you go home and you do any additional research, go on Facebook, or just take charge of your health by going and [then] ask them, "Can this drug do xyz or have this effect?" then they feel you feel you is the doctor now. They see this as an insult to their knowledge [*laughs*] and I am saying, "Well, this happens in North America!" With no problem you can talk to your doctor and say, "Well, I've read this and I'm worried and such." Doesn't matter, every time they give me a drug I does go and research it [*laughs*].

NICOLE: Laypeople have a lot more access to information nowadays.

DAVID: Yes, and traditionally that is not how it was with doctors and patients. But yeah, we're not giving [the vaccine] to my daughter.

As if responding to Nurse Alleyne's suggestion that parents might lack education and simply take what they read online to be as certain as "gospel," David insists that it is because he is prudent and discerning that he takes advantage of his access to online research to find out more about the possible side effects and interactions of any drugs he or his family is prescribed. Outlining the power of the internet to question the totality of biomedical knowledge, he claims its real danger lies less in the fake news and parents' inability to decipher the truth and more in the challenges it poses to biomedical knowledge as uncontestable truth.

Cognizant of the widespread circulation of fake news and pseudoscience on the internet, Afro-Barbadian mothers like Bernadette similarly maintained that the internet was a beneficial place to research the HPV vaccine. When I asked how she responded to medical practitioners' concerns about the danger of blindly relying on the internet, she described the internet as just one of many sources to which she turned when deciding whether to vaccinate her daughter: "I mean, yeah, well I know people who are suspicious because they're like oh conspiracy theorists, or they're crazy, or they're looking for someone to blame and all of these things and that's not the case here. I'm a person who's done a lot of research and not just online, I was reading books that were recommended by lots of different sources to come to my own conclusion." Much in the way David did, Bernadette expressed suspicion toward the medical community's cautionary tales about the internet and Facebook groups online:

I do think that the medical field and with vaccines especially, it's like, if you speak against it, like it's a religion in a way. It's very God-like and it's almost like, "How dare you speak against or question this God-like umm entity in the world. You're not a doctor, you're not a professional!" Yeah, it's almost like sacrilege to just speak out against it in any way or to share your negative experiences and I think that's a problem. And you know, we are in a new information age and we can find out things for ourselves. We need to be careful and do it in the right ways and not believe everything we see and read, but we should be allowed to question people and that's how doctors will become better, when they have to answer those questions in a real way instead of just, "I said so," so, I think [online research] is a new thing worldwide that we have to address.

Inherent in these claims is the belief that the internet is potentially dangerous not because of the misinformation it undoubtedly contains but because of the challenges it poses to medical knowledge which confidently upholds vaccination as protection and nurses and doctors as protectors for disseminating technical medical advice and authority. Indeed, accompanying many professionals' valid concerns about fake news and their frequent conflation of antivaccination propaganda and suspicion is a belief in the certainty of biomedical knowledge and of vaccination as an uncontestable form of protection.

Curiously, despite their certainty about the dangers of the internet and steadfast communication to parents that they should rely exclusively on their biomedical knowledge and expertise, Barbadian doctors and nurses also relied on the internet and social media to promote the HPV vaccine. For instance, in the campaign mentioned in chapter 2, which was promoted by Dr. Chatrani, a prominent obstetrician and gynecologist on Facebook and Instagram as part of the Gyn-A-Thon Barbados initiative, Barbadian parents are encouraged to #GetYourDaughtersVaccinated. In this campaign, vaccination is framed as the responsible choice and the "likable" choice, the shareable, retweetable, popular choice to which online users could rally behind. Campaigns like these, alongside the authorized circulation of viral productions like memes in local polyclinics, suggest the internet's use value not just for the validation and circulation of parents' suspicions but for the circulation of biomedical knowledge and certainty.[14] The use of the internet appears contradictory if not suspicious to Barbadian parents because of the certainty with which these doctors and nurses consistently declare the internet a dangerous place filled with fake news, antivaccination rhetoric, and disinformation about the HPV vaccine. Moreover, through this process, the tenuous concept of certainty and its relationship to suspicion are called into question.

(Biomedical) Certainty and Suspicion

The antonym of hesitation, the term *certainty* refers to truth, fact, assuredness, and absence of doubt.[15] Positioning themselves as the vanguards of biomedical truth, doctors and nurses stressed to me the importance of projecting a sense of certainty about the dangers of HPV, the scientific efficacy of vaccination, and the ills of the internet to mitigate or override parents' suspicions. Despite this and their use of the internet to promote the HPV vaccine, my interviews with public health practitioners further reveal that they harbored some of the same doubts and suspicions for which they counseled patients. In effect, their comments expose how suspicion circulates alongside certainty in the medical establishment— attaching at once to the internet, particular medical professionals, and at times to the vaccine itself.

Dr. Jones was one of the private physicians I interviewed about his views on the HPV vaccine and its dissemination in Barbados through the national program. At the time of our discussion, the Ministry of Health was still offering the vaccine in secondary schools exclusively to young women. Dr. Jones's comments encapsulate the simultaneous expressions of suspicion and certainty uttered by doctors and nurses and echo the open criticism I observed each group presenting toward each other about their respective roles in influencing parents' hesitancy and low uptake of the vaccine:

> It is something new and the Barbadian public is extremely cautious. . . . Right now there is a pushback to anything with a vaccine, so it might just be the time we are in. There was also the cost issue for us, right? It's only been within the last couple weeks that the ministry is selling the vaccine to private doctors for us to give within our private practices. Other than that, we had to bring it in privately and it was something like US$200 a dose which made it extremely prohibitive. And because we weren't able to offer it much in private practice, word sort of got around that only the ministry is offering this and not private doctors because they know something or have a problem with it. So, even though we were saying, "No, there's no problem with it, it's a matter of cost," the public was seeing that we weren't giving it and making their own interpretations. Many people are also getting information either on Facebook or some other nonedited opinion sources that are not helpful in disseminating the facts. The ministry did try to circumvent this with a campaign that was frankly a little dry and noninteresting, and then we had guidance counselors and teachers in secondary school who I thought should have known better but who didn't have the correct information and were

put in the poor position of counseling parents. And then also I think we had unprepared nurses go out there to the target audience. And [some nurses] themselves probably weren't comfortable with the vaccine. . . . When the patients and parents asked pertinent, sensitive questions and nurses faltered with their response, then the hesitancy grew. The intelligent parents asked questions to their own doctors. . . . Personally, I am all for it. I don't know if I would have been for it when it first came out and they jumped on marketing this without the evidence, but now we've had a long enough experience with it, we have seen that there aren't any serious side effects and I have no reservations other than I think it should be given to boys and girls. And I share this with my patients in a very nonpushy, confident manner. I don't put pressure on them; we can always revisit the conversation.

By positioning himself as confident and assertive and nurses as hesitant in their responses to parents, Dr. Jones enfolds nurses into the language of suspicion that surrounds and exists beyond the vaccine. Other doctors with whom I spoke argued that immunization nurses received less than ideal levels of training at the outset of the campaign's rollout and suggested it was their alleged hesitancy to which parents gravitated. As one doctor at the Ministry of Health confirmed,

We did a lot of training, we even had a doctor from overseas come and do training, and we had help from the vaccine company . . . the pharmaceutical company who manufactures the vaccine. . . . They sent in a doctor to help us with the education of both the nurses and the doctors. But it wasn't enough. We did more training of the nurses last year and made sure that it was the nurses who were stronger who were giving the presentations to parents because that didn't happen in 2014 and there were negative consequences for sure. But we doubled our coverage from 2014 to 2015 and I'm sure we will have good coverage in 2016 because we addressed this key issue.

Ironically, this very decision on the part of the ministry to select "strong" nurses to promote the vaccine was what many nurses objected to and felt created more unease in the public. As Nurse Dobbs reflected:

You know, I think if nurses were more involved, well . . . they were involved. I shouldn't say more involved; they were part of the town hall meetings, but it was a selected group of nurses who were chosen to speak to the public, right? And if parents had questions they were directed to those specific few nurses who were speaking about it and I think that that gave the public some measure of suspicion in and of itself because like I said before, with all the other vaccines we introduce, we didn't do all this and like I said, you know, in this society if you have a select group and only those persons are doing it then everyone is like, "Why only them . . . where are the others?"

Echoing Nurse Dobbs, other immunizations nurses with whom I spoke (and whom doctors criticized for appearing hesitant about the vaccine) implicated local and foreign doctors from the Pan American Health Organization in influencing Barbadian parents' suspicion. For these nurses, it was doctors' insistence to spearhead the vaccination program and promote it via the media, town hall meetings, and pharmaceutical advertisements that created unnecessary hype and warranted public skepticism. According to Nurse Alleyne, it was doctors' insistence on spearheading the HPV vaccination campaign and their lack of confidence and experience in doing so that damaged the initiative from the start:

> There were doctors and nurses [who] were adamant that they were not giving it to their own daughters. Some said they wanted to see more research on it and questioned, "Why now, this HPV vaccine?" What I found is, I went to the private international school here, the Codrington School, and most of those kids had already been given the vaccine in their home countries because most of them are diplomats' children and in their birth country Gardasil is one of the vaccines like any other vaccines, so the receptiveness was naturally better. So when we went there we found out well a lot of kids had already had their courses of the vaccine, but here in the other schools, I find that because some health professionals have a mindset against it, they don't, they not pushing it. And in this society, people tend to listen to doctors more than nurses so if the doctors were 100 percent on board in selling it that would have helped in a big way as well. But as I said, the first mistake they made was not to allow us as public health nurses to introduce it. We introduced hepatitis B and such and the parents were receptive because we spoke to them at their level. Yes, everything has side effects, low-grade fever, tenderness at the injection site. Of course, we know as health professionals there are always anomalies, but you do not tell the ordinary man on the street about the anomalies, you know? That is going to give him a negative impact and once you tell him that, he is going to tell his friend who will tell his friend and it mushrooms out. So you give him the basics. . . . The odds of somebody having an anaphylactic shock is very, very minimal. So why are you going to scare off a hundred people telling them about the different things that could go wrong. . . . That creates mass hysteria.

Concerned with doctors' ineffective counseling and what she perceived as the overly forthcoming nature of some nurse practitioners, Nurse Alleyne offers insight into the multiple suspicions that exist in the medical profession. While the nurses and doctors with whom I spoke were unified in critiquing parents' misinformed beliefs and online activities as the main drivers behind suspicion, such comments inadvertently reveal that the binary they often projected between suspicion and biomedical certainty is, in reality, more tenuous than it appears. Indeed, as the excerpts make clear, alongside medical professionals' espoused certainty about parents' lack of internet literacy, the efficacy of the vaccine and their biomedical training are deep-seated suspicions about each other and the degree of certainty and strength in public outreach that each was presumed to have.

Although unspoken to the wider public, the suspicions that doctors and nurses held for each other were palpable to many of the parents with whom I spoke. Reflecting on the apparent inconsistencies she saw between the medical information she was receiving from doctors, public health nurses, and her online research, Harriet exasperatedly claimed, "I saw online that even one of the doctors involved in the creation or testing of the vaccines had worries and concerns about the vaccine and well of course that worried me. So like when I tried to ask the nurse in the polyclinic questions about the vaccine and about this doctor online she didn't have much info, and way back when I asked the nurses at the town hall some questions and they couldn't answer things fully that left me thinking, Well, this really needs to be researched more fully." Parents like Harriet call into question medical certainty's infallibility and the prescribed irrationality of parents' suspicions. The doctor she refers to is Dr. Diane Harper, former consultant for Merck and principal investigator in clinical trials for Gardasil. Over the past decade, Harper's comments about the vaccine have been quoted and misquoted by vaccine promoters and antivaccine groups alike. Hailed as a whistleblower by some for highlighting the unknown long-term efficacy of the vaccine, Harper's words have been misconstrued across many popular online forums in support of the argument that Merck is withholding dangerous information from its consumers.[16] Rather than discrediting the HPV vaccine, as commonly claimed, Harper has instead highlighted the limitations of protection it offers in light of limited long-term efficacy and immunogenicity data. These claims, as published in peer-reviewed scientific research articles by Harper, are supported by cost-effective analyses that suggest that if the three-dose vaccine fails to protect against the specific HPV strains it targets for at least fifteen years, then cervical cancer will only be postponed rather than prevented.[17] Harper has also noted the challenges of complying with the three-dose schedule in many developing countries and maintained that prevention of cervical cancer must continue to rely on screening alongside vaccination. For parents like Harriet, who were seeking clarity on Harper's comments, it was nurses' lack of certainty in their responses to her questions that cemented her decision to forgo the vaccine for her children.

Jacinta, a forty-nine-year-old Afro-Barbadian mother of two who refused the vaccine for her daughter, similarly spoke about the inconsistencies between the claims she was exposed to online and the information (and perceived lack thereof) the Barbadian public health practitioners were providing to the public. Laying out three of the factors she deemed to cement her decision to refuse the vaccine, she said:

> One: It's how it was delivered to me. Two: The way the ministry talked about it, they never talked about side effects. They talked about the glorified benefits but no side effects. And one of the town halls I attended, someone asked about the side effects and the nurse just glossed over the side effects and I'm like but this is so different from what I'm seeing online. . . . I'm seeing death and serious lifelong effects. Three: If this vaccine is not mandatory that means to me, like, it's not really all that transformative and as super as they making it seem, otherwise they'd make it mandatory. Why is what you are saying so different from what we are seeing online? We are seeing images in online support groups of beautiful sixteen-year-old girls who are now vegetables after having the vaccine. And some parents hadn't even seen these videos, but they heard about it and that was enough to make them concerned. And in response the nurses are telling us that things are different now from when we were growing up and that now our kids are highly sexualized and the vaccine is beneficial. But I don't agree with that. I was suspicious, that's the truth. Caribbean people are naturally suspicious.

Bringing awareness to what she felt was hesitancy from doctors and nurses to disclose all possible information on the vaccine, Jacinta questions not only their honesty in disclosing the vaccine's side effects to the Barbadian public but their breadth of knowledge about its efficacy and ultimately its necessity. Framing her disillusionment with the vaccine in terms of the discrepancies she noted between doctors' and nurses' counseling and the viral videos she was exposed to online, Jacinta asserts suspicion as that which exists in contrast to and in the absence of certainty. While the doctors and nurses I detail herein similarly position suspicion as oppositional and, at best, inversely related to biomedical certainty, doing so overlooks the possible simultaneity, fallibility, and generativity of suspicion and certainty and further perpetuates this untenable binary between them. Indeed, though many of these same medical professionals fixated on the role their colleagues' certainty (or lack thereof) had in influencing parents' suspicion, they also defeatedly revealed their own ambivalences toward the HPV vaccine.

Temporarily removing their medical hats, doctors and nurses often surprised me by casually sharing their suspicions about the vaccine as Barbadian parents and citizens themselves. As mentioned in chapter 4, many of the medical professionals I interviewed spoke emphatically about the need for doctors and nurses to frame the vaccine as something that protects against cervical cancer rather than the sexually transmitted infection of HPV. For Dr. Pack, this strategy was fundamental for encouraging the average patient to understand the vaccine's cruciality and to mitigate suspicion about its relationship to adolescent sex. When I asked if he could empathize at all with parents' sense of hesitancy around the vaccine despite the seriousness and severity of cervical cancer in the developing world, he responded, "Well of course, I don't know many people who aren't ambivalent. . . . I'm even a little ambivalent because it's relatively recently introduced compared to the others . . . but it's clear that this vaccine is one of the best chances we have of reducing cervical cancer rates in the region." Within seconds of revealing his own ambivalence, Dr. Pack changed the topic and proceeded to share one of the slides he used during presentations he gave to communities of parents in an effort to foreground the irrationality that he believed to constitute citizens' resistance to the vaccine. He said wryly, "So one of my slides which may be a little bit offensive but that I use is, 'THERE'S NO VACCINE AGAINST STUPIDITY.' But I'm not calling anybody stupid, right? I just put it up there for a quick second and then take it down." By suggesting that his slide is meant to be tongue-in-cheek, Dr. Pack seeks to downplay the thinly veiled but common perception among medical professionals of parents who are hesitant, are suspicious, or refuse vaccination as irrational, ignorant, and uninformed. As I detailed in chapter 4, such a characterization and subsequent dismissal of parents' suspicious sensibilities fails to account for the embodied, instinctual, and enfleshed theories through which many Barbadian parents are reasoning to refuse vaccination and, in so doing, offer a different, fraught form of protection to their children. Moreover, as is apparent in Dr. Pack's statements, while certainty and confidence in the biomedical sensibility of vaccination as the primary mode of protection against HPV exist closely alongside a condemnation of suspicion and refusal, they also exist in tandem with a range of suspicions, uncertainties, contradictions, and ambivalences held by Barbadian doctors and nurses about the HPV vaccine.

So widespread were doctors' and nurses' personal and often undisclosed uncertainties about the vaccine, Nurse Pitt shared, she had trouble conceiving a smooth rollout of the vaccination program:

I have to say I already envisioned the problem at the onset. To be frank, I had my own personal reservations based on the fact that generally when we are going to provide vaccines to the public, it goes through a longer period of testing and I thought that in some ways the pharmaceutical company was not straightforward in terms of information even to providers, furthermore to the public. Because first they said that they tested the thing for five years, then now you heard that it was only tested for three years and I thought you know, if we are going to be administering vaccines or any form of medication, especially when it's the unknown, then it should go through a long-term study of at least ten years. I would say I felt comfortable to a certain point, and I say a certain point because I was still guarded. . . . Many of my colleagues too were extremely reticent. Some of them refused to give the vaccine to their own, they would smile and say yes when other parents asked if they would [agree to the vaccine for their children], but even some of those who were involved with the promotion through the ministry, they refused to give the vaccine to their children. So I respected the ministry's effort, but you know again I think many were guarded. . . . Even those [officials] on top, I think they were guarded. And it was under the excuse that we didn't have enough funds that the ministry kept saying, you know, we will just vaccinate x amount of people right now and only girls at the beginning but I think that shows they were being precautious. I mean knowing that cancer is a horrible disease and can metastasize and at times I did think, Well, wow, if this can be prevented I should be for it. And knowing that most of our breadwinners are single women, about 65 percent of our households are female headed . . . and I thought, well, no, okay we have something that can prevent cancer for these women, and I think that made me gain some more confidence in providing the vaccine. And in my experience, I've seen no child develop an adverse reaction. When the ministry decided to offer it to boys and to the class 4s I was relieved right, because at first parents would be wondering, Why only girls? You want to kill out our girls or what? So I was relieved when the program expanded because when I was doing my presentations I had to calm parents by saying, "We nurses really don't want to see pregnant preteens or teenagers in this polyclinic." I said, "We have enough work to do and I personally don't need that hassle, so you know, we don't have any hidden agenda that your child be more promiscuous, we are just trying to protect your child."

Nurse Pitt fluctuates between expressing the warranted suspicions she and her colleagues held about the vaccine, the sense of shame she nonetheless felt for having these suspicions, and the promises the vaccine offered young Barbadians (particularly young women) to protect against cervical cancer.

Nurse Sobers similarly reflected on her positionality as both a nurse and an Afro-Barbadian mother who championed the vaccine at work but struggled privately to reconcile its association with sex with the benefits it promised young women: "One of the main issues for parents was that the vaccine somehow seemed to be related to sex and once the vaccine was given, I think parents were a bit concerned that their child would then start having sexual intercourse. And for us, for us parents in the Caribbean, we don't talk about sex, right. We don't talk about sex, so the fact that it was related to sex was a major challenge for parents to deal with." Like the medical professionals I interviewed over the course of this research, Nurse Sobers relayed what she believed to be parents' concerns over the HPV vaccine because of its connections to adolescent sex. Yet by claiming that "for *us* parents" there was an unmistakable relationship between the HPV vaccine and sex, she is clear that she occupies multiple identities and spaces. Using the pronoun *us*, she oscillates between representing the Ministry of Health whose aim is to encourage parents to vaccinate their children and her identity as an Afro-Barbadian mother who claims to have been socialized in a certain cultural repertoire that believes sex is a taboo subject. Like Jacinta, who states, "Caribbean people are naturally suspicious," she importantly draws attention to a commonly overlooked shared identity among the parents, doctors, and nurses and parents who are doctors or nurses who make these various claims about suspicion and certainty.

Danielle chose to accept the HPV vaccine for her eldest daughter despite her lingering suspicions. She was struck at the dismissal not simply of parents' suspicion but of what she believed was a shared sense of Caribbeanness between Barbadian laypeople and medical professionals:

> The people trying to discredit what we parents were reading online aren't necessarily doing the best job. That's really a problem. At my daughter's school we had a doctor come in and I didn't get to ask anything because there were so many questions but I am not even sure that speaking to one of them would have eased my mind because they are so biased. The same doctor who was there said, "I know y'all going on the internet and seeing all this foolishness!" And I thought, "Listen, do not disregard parents' feelings." My feelings and concerns are real to me and when you have someone in the medical profession thinking only about science, that is not a Caribbean thing. People

in the Caribbean who don't believe in God still have a spirituality attached to their lives, and to disregard feelings and emotions and spiritual beliefs that come along with parenting and protecting your children really turned me off. Science doesn't have all the answers and at the very least, you have to respect our ways of understanding this and our concerns.

By connecting a sense of spirituality to Barbadian parents' feelings of uncertainty, skepticism, and suspicion and differentiating these emotions from scientific claims to rationality and objectivity, assertions like Danielle's support my argument surrounding suspicion's cultural and affective resonance for Afro-Barbadians and further emphasize the complex, divergent, and overlapping subjectivities that suspicion (and certainty) engender for differently situated Barbadians.

Contextualizing suspicion in a Caribbean identity that is attuned to the erotic, the divine, and the sacred, both Danielle and Nurse Sobers gesture to what Arlie Hochschild has called "feeling rules"—prescribed beliefs that dictate the affective feelings, emotions, and norms expected of people in different social, cultural, economic, and occupational contexts.[18] As Hochschild notes, in guiding the recognition and legitimation of feelings, cultures often engender and lay out the possibilities for different subjectivities in spoken and unspoken ways and support their emergent narrative frameworks.[19] As this book has illustrated, suspicion is a distributed affective form that circulates for Afro-Barbadians in the various socioeconomic, political, and historical formations that contextualize technologies like the HPV vaccine, the adolescents (and adolescent sex) whom these technologies target, the government's precarious economy, growing assemblages of multinational pharmaceutical networks, and, to a significant extent, longer transnational histories of slavery, capitalist extraction, and public health in the anglophone Caribbean. As the Afro-Barbadian parents herein highlight, suspicion subsequently affects and shapes their engagements with technologies like the vaccine, as well as their relationship to biomedical, pharmaceutical, and governmental claims to knowledge about certainty, hesitancy, and the protection the vaccine claims to provide. For differently situated Barbadian doctors and nurses with whom I spoke, however, feeling rules in the medical profession appeared to distinctly dictate a sense of comfort and certainty in science and biotechnologies like the HPV vaccine alongside a sense of gratitude for the privilege to access such medical interventions. Such rules, as parents like Jacinta and Harriet argued, curiously preclude affects and norms like caution, skepticism, spirituality, and suspicion that circulate in Barbadian culture writ large and perceivably do so across intersections of race, class, gender, and occupation. As the excerpts from medical professionals show, despite and amid their certainties and projections of confidence in the vaccine, they often simultaneously experience suspicion and skepticism as they counsel parents and promote the vaccine. By no means limited to the beliefs of medical professionals, Afro-Barbadian parents like Danielle who did accept the HPV vaccine held a similar a sense of confidence and certainty in the technology of the vaccine and the protection it could offer their child, and this existed alongside a sense of suspicion. Although not the focus of this study, such parents' voices in conversation with confessionary narratives such as Nurse Pitt's, Nurse Sobers's and Dr. Pack's variously illustrate the simultaneity of certainty and suspicion for differently situated Barbadians, and the (ironic) fallibility of certainty—its inevitable liability to doubt, tentativeness, and unreliability.

Elizabeth is another parent who accepted the vaccine for her daughter and yet responded to my call to interview parents who were ambivalent about it. A white Bajan mother of three who requested that her fourteen-year-old daughter Tara receive the vaccine when it was first introduced by the Ministry of Health in 2014, Elizabeth's story weaves together these sensibilities of certainty and suspicion and their inevitable shortcomings. She remembered being eager to act quickly at the first chance she got to protect her daughter from cervical cancer, and after consulting with Tara's private pediatrician, arrangements were made for her to receive the first of three shots. When I asked her if she had any qualms about the vaccine at that time she responded, "Um, no, we, we vaccinate. We do what the pediatrician tells us to do [*laughs*] and that, ah, sounds simplistic [*laughs*] but we've never not immunized, or not done [what was advised], we've never had any issues with the advice the pediatrician has given us regarding the medical path. We do . . . we are a healthy household."

Over the course of an hour, Elizabeth relayed the dramatic events that unfolded in the days and months after Tara's first dosage of the vaccine. Within two days, she recalled, her daughter developed flu-like symptoms, including severe headaches, body aches, and fever. By the third day, a rash had developed, and Elizabeth noticed increased fatigue, listlessness, and crying. Tara was "just a miserable, very, very unhappy child," she recalled. At that point, Elizabeth and her husband sought medical attention at a nearby private medical hospital, where a team of doctors eventually diagnosed and treated Tara for a viral illness over the course of about six weeks. At no point before or during her observation at the hospital was a connection made between her symptoms and the HPV vaccine, by either doctors or Elizabeth and her husband. Upon her discharge from the hospital, Tara returned to school but struggled to catch up on all she had missed during her lengthy absence. As Elizabeth notes,

The school was very supportive, but Tara couldn't cope in a number of ways, especially emotionally, she went on sort of a downward emotional spiral. Yeah, she couldn't cope. So that then mushroomed into a whole, ah, diagnosis of emotional and mental disorder where she was then diagnosed with depression and anxiety which was probably, possibly genetically there, but I believe came out with this drama, as I believe genetic things, I think do. . . . We ended up moving her from her prestigious secondary school and thankfully we were able to reenroll her in the private school that she came out of . . . and there was then stress associated with that, adolescence, resocializing, etc. All the while she continued with headaches, up until to today she still gets severe headaches.

During our interview, which took place a year and a half after her "nightmare," began, Elizabeth reflected on her prior enthusiasm to accept the vaccine in light of Tara's host of new medical conditions, questioning her uncritical adherence to medical advice and the protection the vaccine promised to offer:

ELIZABETH: We know a number of her peers in the school and in other schools, whose parents opted not to immunize their children and I was like, "You're kidding! You have an opportunity to protect your child and you're not?" And look what happened to me! Look what happened! Life goes on. Obviously, the polyclinic and the Ministry of Health, they all agreed with me that they did not recommend that we continue with the other two dosages.

NICOLE: And this was true even though they didn't acknowledge a direct correlation between her symptoms and the vaccine?

ELIZABETH: Correct. Yep, yep. It was risky, they say now, and her pediatrician agreed with that too. But to this day they do not and will not acknowledge that her rapid onset of these symptoms is directly related to the vaccine. The pediatrician was quite adamant with me, "No, Elizabeth, na, na, na, na." I said, "We will agree to disagree."

NICOLE: And so do you think or feel differently about the vaccine now? Do you think your situation and experience was just one in a million?

ELIZABETH: I think that my situation has to be one in a million, yes. I have said nothing negative to anyone else. If a parent approached me and asked me a question I will share my experience. I would not go out, go about and advocate people do not immunize against it. I, well, how do I think about it now? I am convinced that her illness was associated with the vaccine. I mean, we took her to a neurologist who diagnosed her with migraines. Um, it is not my belief that she had migraines at all. It is my belief that [and] coinciding with what I have read now online where these children's symptoms go on for years after the vaccine, it is my belief this is still part of the HPV vaccine's side effects. Because [the symptoms] are getting further apart. Could she have had a bad dose, or vial? I guess. I am not convinced that the vaccine is a bad thing though. And I don't feel negative towards the ministry or the school or the system or the medical fraternity for offering the vaccine. No, the only sadness I have is what we had to undergo.

NICOLE: And now, after your experiences, do you view those parents who might have been ambivalent or who had concerns about perceived side effects in a different light? You mentioned that prior to this experience you thought, "How could you *not* want to protect your child?"

ELIZABETH: I do. Yeah, I do. I ... [*sigh*], I ... I guess I commend [those parents] for not just blindly listening to expert people, medical experts. Because for me it was and still, I'm thinking like but, how do you *not* listen to your doctor? But you should, you should question, you should check. If I had to live again and do it again, I wouldn't take blind advice. So if in ten years' time a cancer vaccine becomes available and I have the opportunity to vaccinate my child and myself, I will not blindly go and have it or give my child. I will attempt to do research on it. And that's how [this experience] has changed my view. Because if I had known at the beginning what I know at the end, I may have not immunized her.

We can trace how Elizabeth's understanding of protection expands as a result of her daughter's negative experiences, which she firmly attributes to the vaccine. While at first she critiques the decision of fellow Barbadian parents to refuse the vaccine, baffled at how one could choose against protecting children and dismiss the professional opinions and certainty of the medical fraternity, she has begun to understand the significance of some parents' gut sensibilities and suspicions toward the vaccine. Turning to social media and the internet to conduct research only after her daughter received the vaccine, Elizabeth inserts herself into the same transnational affective online communities that parents throughout this book do, noting that they now offer her support and validate her daughter's painful and traumatic experiences in a way doctors have been unable to.

Though Elizabeth also told me, "We stopped her after the first dose, hence she's not protected," a sense of empathy and affectivity between other parents' multiple suspicions and concerns about the vaccine has arguably altered Elizabeth's current sense of the multiplicity of protection and certainty. That is, she has come to appreciate and "commend" others for embodying and theorizing an ethics of protection that transcends the superiority of biomedical certainty and biomedical sensibilities of protection from cervical cancer through vaccination. As detailed in chapter 4, through suspicion and a refusal of the vaccine, many of the Afro-Barbadian parents I interviewed over the course of this research expressed and embodied a fraught understanding of protection from the vaccine's unknown side effects, from incidental pain and suffering, government neglect, pharmaceutical interests, the dangerous hegemony of a biopolitics of care, and for some the psychic pain and memories of force and control of Black women under slavery. Elizabeth's commitment to no longer blindly accept medical advice echoes that of Nurse Jane, frustrated at parents' blind adherence to what they view online, and gets at the crux of these multiple constitutions of suspicion, certainty, and protection. Why has a responsible parent been framed as one who unquestionably follows medical advice, certainty, and knowledge? How might we appreciate the multiple sensibilities of suspicion and certainty that inhere in understandings of protection while remaining cognizant of their limitations?

Elizabeth's experiences recall the anxieties expressed by mothers like Naitry and Bee discussed in chapter 4 whose deep concerns about the potential side effects of the vaccine on their daughters' lives had a tenacious hold on their decision making about the vaccine and who collectively mused about who would suffer should something go seriously wrong. "Who will stay home with my ailing daughter while I must work? How will this affect our financial stability?" Bee asked. As Elizabeth reflects and believes, Tara is now one such seriously affected child, and she, a parent, is burdened with arranging for her mental and physical care.

Although we can trace how affects of suspicion attach to Barbadians like Elizabeth in the wake of her negative experiences, her story undeniably underscores the influence of race and class in thinking through the subtleties and variations in these epistemologies of suspicion and certainty. Elizabeth is a well-off white woman with an upper-management job in a large company. Her concerns about Tara's health do not extend to questions about money, government assistance, the financial stakes of caretaking, or histories of colonial medical injustice and experimentation toward and on Black people in the Caribbean. Not only did she note that she and her family always ate healthy (and organic) foods when available, she arranged for Tara to see a number of private specialists, from psychiatrists to neurologists, to cover "all aspect[s] of [Tara's] challenge." When she first became ill, Tara was taken to a nearby private health facility, where she received intensive and undoubtedly costly medical care. When Tara was unable to reintegrate into her public school, Elizabeth and her husband could afford for her to reenter the private school she had previously attended.

I offer sustained attention to Elizabeth's story for two reasons. First, despite her experiences and resulting sense of empathy toward parents' suspicions about the vaccine, Elizabeth does not and perhaps cannot articulate affects of suspicion as the Afro-Barbadian parents I have interviewed throughout this book have.

It is notable that despite her emerging sense of the multiple subjectivities, feelings, and constitutions of protection that surround the complicated question of HPV vaccination uptake, and her growing sense of empathy (as a parent) toward other Barbadian parents who refused the vaccine, she is clear to note she has no ill feeling or distrust toward the Ministry of Health, the government, or her pediatrician, with whom she strongly disagrees about the cause of Tara's sudden and extensive list of medical conditions. As an upper-class white Barbadian, Elizabeth's sustained faith in the government, the medical community, and even the pharmaceutical product Gardasil, which she's "not convinced . . . is a bad thing," exists in stark contrast to the many Afro-Barbadian parents for whom legacies of biopolitical and necropolitical care related to the medical institution weigh heavy as residue. By vernacularly reframing hesitancy as suspicion, Afro-Barbadians tell of the persistent histories of colonialism and capitalism in the anglophone Caribbean, of which science and medicine are an integral part.

As I have argued in conversation with women of color, Black, and transnational feminist theorists of affect, for many such parents, suspicion and protection are theories and understandings that emerge through the flesh, through gut feelings, affective memories, racialized and palimpsestic sensibilities of force, and distrust around the vaccine. For these Afro-Barbadian parents, suspicion surfaced significantly in relation to what they perceived to be the government's allegiance to the transnational medicopharmaceutical industry, questionable interests in the health and vitality of Barbadians, and the notion of protection it promoted. By emphasizing her belief that her daughter is "not protected" from HPV and cervical cancer because she failed to receive the full dosage of the vaccine, Elizabeth refuses these understandings of suspicion and protection, accentuating the racial dimensions of suspicion and connected forms of biopolitical refusals which the Afro-Barbadian parents in this book have outlined.

Second, Elizabeth's experiences, like the revelations and omissions by the Barbadian medical professionals with whom I spoke, offer further clarity and insight into the sensibility of certainty as fraught, defensive, and imperfect. To recognize this is to let go of the artificial and untenable binary so often upheld between suspicion and certainty that paints suspicion as an irrational mode of resistance in contrast to the rational, autonomous, and objective truths of biomedical knowledge and certainty. Certainty's likelihood to be erroneous, subject to change, and even false is especially significant in light of medical professionals' investment in discrediting the fake news, disinformation, and unverifiable literature online with which I began this chapter and which doctors and nurses often assumed underlaid parents' suspicion. Unlike the stance of biomedical certainty, affects like suspicion exist beyond the rationality/irrationality and truth/post-truth binaries. At a time when the media, politics, and public health are facing an arguable crisis of truth, it is crucial that we seek to understand how affective intensities like suspicion operate not just counter to but alongside and within realms like public health. As chapter 4 gestured toward, appreciating suspicion recognizes its emotional appeals for Afro-Barbadians in spite of its many potentially fraught implications for their health outcomes. Furthermore, as this chapter details, reckoning with suspicion acknowledges certainty's fallibility and accepts the uncertainty, injurious history, imperfection, and risk that equally informs theoretical biomedicine, its technologies, and the biomedical knowledge that medical professionals universally and defensively uphold as unequivocal truth. Coming to terms with certainty as fallible means releasing investments in suspicion as the purely (negative) antithesis of certainty, turning away from the embattled narratives between the two and accepting suspicion and certainty as generative in spite of their inescapable shortcomings. Like risk and care in the history of Barbados and the anglophone Caribbean, we must recognize suspicion and certainty to exist in a symbiotic, circular, and frustratingly fraught dynamic through which both sensibilities and their emergent subjectivities are continually restructured. Recognizing this is vital to public health efforts that seek to address vaccine hesitancy in different locations and in relation to specific vaccines. In the context of HPV vaccination in Barbados, the history of feminist health care activism in the Caribbean around reproductive tract infections and cervical cancer offers generative insight into how the mechanics of public health campaigns that recognize this and work alongside communal residues and affects of suspicion might operate.

Certainty and Suspicion in Health Organizing

Education is doomed to failure when it does not take cultural and social factors into account. This has been seen, for example, in efforts to educate people in family planning. Another element to be considered is *who* is being educated. A simple increase in the number of prepared professional personnel does not, in itself, answer all health needs. — NITA BARROW, "Women in the Front Line of Health Care" (1980)

In August 1978, the Women and Development Unit (WAND) was established by a group of Caribbean feminist scholars and activists with the aim of promoting women's health issues through a participatory model of education and activism. Alongside nongovernmental organizations, WAND members (including Barbadian nurse and humanitarian Dame Nita Barrow, Grenadian-born Peggy Antrobus, and the late Guyanese grassroots feminist Andaiye) engaged with communities' concerns through participatory action research, critiqued the inadequacy of biomedical models of care for Afro-Caribbean women, and modeled more effective forms of disease prevention across community and national levels.

Following a 1992 meeting held in Barbados on reproductive tract infections among women in the Third World, Andaiye and WAND members prepared a feminist political campaign to foreground the injurious economic and political circumstances that disproportionately shaped sex, sexual health risks, and the availability of health care procedures like Pap smears across Latin America and the Caribbean. Titled "Demystifying and Fighting Cervical Cancer," the campaign drew attention to the damaging transnational political and economic conditions that led places like Barbados to have poor access to Pap smear screening and some of the highest rates of cervical cancer globally.[20] WAND critiqued the increasing deployment of Pap screening as a tool of "empowerment" for women, noting it was implicitly bound up in global capital and neoliberalism. The campaign sought to remap the discussion of cervical cancer screening in terms of race, class, imperialism, and embodiment. In so doing, WAND envisioned new forms of transnational networks and epistemologies of care and protection for women in the Global South and called attention to how poverty, poor diet, gender inequality, environmental pollution, environmental racism, and injustice were disproportionally affecting these regions. Significantly, the campaign traced connections between these social ills and rising rates of cancers of the mouth, liver, stomach, and cervix in the Global South—cancers that, at the time of publication, were decreasing in the Global North, yet increasing across the "developing" world, leading to their characterization as "cancers of underdevelopment."[21] In the twenty-first century, much remains the same, with cervical cancer unevenly plaguing the regions of Latin America and the Caribbean. While the HPV vaccine purports to intervene significantly in this landscape, larger public health efforts on behalf of the Barbadian state have much to benefit from closer attention to feminist health campaigns, such as WAND's, which was focused on destigmatizing and educating the Caribbean public on cervical cancer, HPV, and its associated diseases.

The campaign reframed the medical language around cervical cancer and its risk factors in culturally relatable and layperson's terms to relay its severity and empower Latin American and Caribbean women to invest in their health. Looking to feminist foremothers in the English-speaking Caribbean region (and in Barbados specifically) who had successfully liaised with local health clinics, used role-playing and poetry, produced grassroots videos on cervical cancer prevention, and conducted "outreach education program[s] at the community level to encourage use of pap smear services," the campaign emphasized the need to share information at the grassroots level to promote preventive services in the long run.[22] This form of feminist organizing, WAND noted, was crucial to combat not only the cervical cancer plaguing the region but the shame and guilt women often felt on being diagnosed with HPV or abnormal cells, a shame often "compounded by the insensitivity of medical personnel" and in other cases by their male spouses or partners.[23] Further modeling their vision of a successful community-oriented health campaign on previous forms of organizing and feminist advocacy against cervical cancer in South Africa, Peru, and Bolivia from the late 1980s and early 1990s, WAND's campaign documented the resonance of community engagement for at-risk women across the developing world. Of specific note was the success of Bolivian women's community members in encouraging women to get Pap smears by disseminating information about cervical cancer in local churches, in community centers, and through door-to-door canvassing and TV commercials, alongside more standardized public health brochures and posters and physicians and gynecologists in hospitals and health care clinics.

As Nita Barrow tirelessly advocated in and across her multiple careers as a public health nurse and activist in Barbados and Jamaica, adviser to the Pan American Health Organization, governor general of Barbados (to name a few of her roles), education, consensus building, and community engagement are necessary for equitable health outcomes because they spread the message about biomedical confidence in health care interventions such as Pap smears and foster trust, self-determination, comfort, and well-being for at-risk women.[24] Nearly three decades later, much remains to be accomplished regarding community health engagement around cervical cancer in Barbados, of which the recent introduction of the HPV vaccine across many English-speaking Caribbean countries is just a part. Many of the Afro-Barbadian mothers with whom I spoke called attention to this, indicating a yearning for a form of medical education around HPV that is sympathetic to the complex valences of suspicion and certainty.

Donna is a thirty-four-year-old Afro-Caribbean massage therapist and mother of two daughters, about one of whom she recently made the decision not to vaccinate with Gardasil. In our interview, Donna expressed skepticism about the HPV vaccine because it was not "tried and true" in the ways that routine childhood immunizations and traditional herbal remedies were in her family's experience:

My youngest daughter is asthmatic so we have all the medications, nebulizers, everything, but we also use natural remedies. So she will eat the "wonder of world" [*Kalanchoe pinnata*] plant, like if she's wheezing she will eat that and it helps clear the mucus from her chest. If that doesn't work, then we will move on to the inhalers. Look, it's understandable that prayer heals and the natural remedies work sometimes, but there are some circumstances where medicine is necessary and I will go ahead and choose that, right. But in this case, we are just being told that there is this vaccine that we need and that's about it. With the old vaccines I know me and my friends all had them, we came up together and we were all fine and nothing out of the ordinary happened. And so I felt my kids could get those too because they had been tried and true and tested. When it came now to this new one that just kind of popped up and the public nurses were casually like, "Oh, we gonna give it to your child!" When I said no to the vaccine I talked to my daughter about it, because a lot of her friends were getting it. A lot of the parents they were just like, "Oh, [the ministry] is offering an extra shot it's fine" and I was like, "But you don't even know what it's for!" Some of these parents only found out about the HPV vaccine the same day they accepted it at the polyclinic. And all the nurses said was that it's just to prevent HPV, but they didn't go in depth in any way. And like I said, I had heard about HPV in my life but never looked into it until I heard about the vaccine after a pharmaceutical ad on TV and then did my research, but the nurses never went into talking about the fact that HPV can come and go spontaneously and lives within you naturally or anything.

Although Donna strongly advocates for traditional herbal remedies as the first course of action for her daughter's health, she incisively acknowledges their limitations and the power of "medicine" in specific situations. Frustrated at the absence of in-depth information from immunization nurses, Donna, like many of the mothers I interviewed, connects her suspicions about the vaccine to the uncertainty that she perceived nurses to have about the vaccine and its efficacy. Although some parents did reflect on the ways they felt they could educate and thus protect their daughters from HPV, more pressing was a desire to protect their children from the plethora of unknowns they felt existed around the vaccine and the forceful and off-putting manner in which it was promoted.

Jacinta encapsulates these multiple efforts to protect her daughter and navigate how the HPV campaign was presented to Afro-Barbadian women like herself:

> With this issue of cervical cancer and HPV, I would give my daughter education about sex and the risks. Even if I am not excited about her being sexually active, I have already said to her, "This is what condoms are for, even for oral sex, there are flavored condoms." I tell her about peer pressure to have sex, about desire, about the body. I am very open, we talk constantly to the point that she gets tired of me talking [*laughs*] but this is how I am choosing to parent and protect her. If I look at my life, or the generation before me, we didn't have a vaccine for this and I'm skeptical that there is a need for this right now it doesn't seem like a life and death situation or circumstance like measles—and the ministry never said it was so severe. And well, I probably would have trusted them more if they had come upfront and presented things in a different way. It's like when my daughter was born, her pediatrician who I knew well was really forthright and explained the different vaccines we would be giving and that they were routinized and tested and he was like, "You probably had all of these yourself." So this information was all given in advance and we had a good rapport, right. And well generally I think Caribbean people have had things come down through our generations about the power of "herbs." For things like common cold, that sort of stuff, I will try a home remedy first and if that didn't work I would go to the doctor because that's how I was taught to manage these things by my mother and so forth—the natural way and through the tradition of them teaching you. Whereas with this vaccine I didn't really feel good about it. Somehow the wording of the forms was very commanding and not personal, and the things on TV it was like, "This is what you need to do," and you can opt out, but like, "[You should] do it." And there wasn't one-on-one information with someone we knew and were comfortable with. I don't know if I'm making sense, but something about it . . . and how we were told about [it] . . . I was like, "No."

Similar to Donna and Jacinta, Natty, a thirty-year-old mother of three children mentioned in chapter 2, refused the vaccine for her eldest son and daughter and invoked traditional health-seeking behaviors and remedies in her discussion of suspicion. According to Natty, it should be obvious to the government that Afro-Caribbean parents are likely to have more faith and trust in fellow community workers than foreign doctors from the Pan American Health Organization when being introduced to "new" viruses like HPV and its recommended preventive vaccine:

> I was raised with a Vincentian mom, so everything is about bush. Bush or menthol crystals and herbs, and still today I go to these remedies first. Even if I go to the doctor, he might prescribe something and I will still use herbal remedies [*laughs*]. I just wanna know what's wrong with me, I want the diagnosis and then I could fix the problem. I think the ways to educate us in the Caribbean about new vaccines and diseases like HPV, being as we are suspicious people, is to get out in neighborhoods, have one-on-ones like how you are interviewing me right now. Talk to people, more community works. I mean, I think you will find it easier to get some of us Bajans to speak to a community member than to attend a town hall with politicians or doctors. So I think they need to rethink this and come out more in different ways and give us the information on HPV and health in a different way that isn't just about trying to convince us about the vaccine alone. And don't wait until [secondary school entrance exams] to spring this on parents. Now that this vaccine is out, we should be learning about it from way before and not just given a form to sign when we come to the clinic out of the blue.

Natty's suspicions do not simply index medical mistrust, but are deeply enveloped with a belief in what health care education should look and feel like—that is, education that is orally transmitted, community-based, and perhaps divorced from attempts to market a pharmaceutical product. Although her subsequently derived ethics to protect her children results in a refusal of the HPV vaccine, it also speaks to a desire to honor Caribbean oral knowledge and health care traditions alongside biomedicine and biomedical knowledge. Often in the same breath, these mothers astutely identified the role of herbs and herbal remedies, the occasional necessity of biomedical interventions, and the more effective ways that they believed doctors and nurses could present pharmaceutical drugs to and increase vaccine compliance among "suspicious people."

The interventions these parents gestured toward align closely with historical visions of Caribbean feminist health care activism formulated in concert with at-risk communities. In describing their suspicions about the vaccine, these parents make known a particular sense of knowing and relating to care rooted in a sense of Caribbeanness—a geographically unbounded, cross-temporal mode of being and a protectiveness that is eternally informed by plantation slavery, colonialism, its fragmentation and migratory circuits, and the enfleshed, embodied, and felt histories of these processes.[25] In contrast to expressing strategic forms of resistance toward the vaccine, Afro-Barbadian parents herein wrestle with these suspicious affects, centuries-long residues, and feeling rules that co-constitute their experiences of biomedicine and their consumption of increasingly common neoliberal, state-biomedical-pharmaceutical campaigns and technologies like the HPV vaccine. Taking seriously parents' claims to knowledge and the sensibility derived from their suspicion is to acknowledge that suspicion is generative of more than refusal. In other words, if hesitancy and suspicion toward the HPV vaccine were seen not as the end points but the beginnings of better health care organizing and organizing in Afro-Caribbean communities in Barbados, new possibilities for biomedical campaigns and the transformation of community health outcomes might emerge.

Although this book's arguments around suspicion and the HPV vaccine center on Barbados and its place in the English-speaking Caribbean, thinking through a transnational feminist framework invites us to trace the heterogeneity and inhabitation of this wariness, sense of knowing and world-making, and specifically the resonance of suspicious affects, "feeling rules," and the related efficacy of community engagement and education around health care in Black communities across the African diaspora. Alondra Nelson's *Body and Soul* poignantly reveals how the Black Panthers in the United States in the late 1960s actively forged and reformulated an understanding of health around social issues—conceiving the then-pervasive commodification of health and health inequity in Black communities as a microcosm of the quotidian forms of racial capitalism and violence in the wake of Jim Crow. Deeply critical of the medical establishment, state-sponsored medical programs, and a "dialect of neglect and surveillance" that seemed to characterize the US landscape for African Americans, the Black Panthers practiced and promoted lay empowerment through health education outreach, training community health care workers by volunteer medical professionals, and establishing community-based clinics.[26] Of great importance was the value the Black Panthers placed on "reducat[ing]" the medical professionals who partnered with them by exposing them to the ideas of Mao Zedong, Frantz Fanon, and other "policy thinkers" who spoke to the transformative potential of lay knowledge for community health and medicine's colonial origins, respectively, all with the intention of creating a dialogue of understanding of the community's historically and contemporary relevant concerns and needs.[27]

Together, the campaigns envisioned by the Black Panthers and WAND activists speak to the historical and productive potential of Black communities' frustration and determination around health care and the urgency of diagnosing the socioeconomic and political inequities around their health. Indicative of suspicion's affective, palimpsestic, traceable indications and M. Jacqui Alexander's generative offering of the operative "here and there" and "then and now" to signal the residual and scrambled qualities of time transnationally, Afro-Barbadian parents invoke suspicion as a response to the political-economic situation in Barbados and to historical legacies and logics of biomedicine and its contentiously perceived state-medical-pharmaceutical economic assemblages—even though the HPV vaccine is being offered to Barbadian citizens free of charge.[28]

Conclusion

Walking to her car after our interview, Harriet turned to me and said, "The government and the health officials have the ability to put stuff out there in a better way that we can feel comfortable, [so] why won't they?" Her words emphasize how a seemingly negative orientation to the vaccine via suspicion is simultaneously optimistic about the future of her children's health and the belief that care and protection can and must be imagined differently. For many of the Afro-Barbadian parents I interviewed, suspicion led to a refusal of the vaccine, but it also opened the door to an imaginative curiosity and, in some cases, a demand for a more active, collective form of community engagement, knowledge translation, and biomedical certainty expressed by the government and its health ministries and associated industries.

As previously noted, the Barbadian Ministry of Health's atypical decision to implement a school-based HPV vaccination program alongside media campaigns, town hall and parent–teacher meetings was modeled after international (predominantly North American and European) research that suggests it to be an effective method of targeting adolescents before they become sexually active and ensuring the multidose completion of the vaccine. Although some nurses speculated that this approach overlooked the cultural politics around sex in Barbados and the wider Caribbean, of greater issue is perhaps its failure to engage and educate local communities in ways that are respectful of and resonant with historical efforts at health care activism around the inequity of cervical cancer in the Caribbean.

As this chapter has shown, overlooking the complexity of suspicion and certainty further constrains possibilities for theoretical or academic investigations into the politics of affect and its complex racialized and gendered valences in contemporary public health campaigns in the anglophone Caribbean. With antiscience viewpoints and disinformation increasingly mischaracterized on a global scale as merely irrational and nonsensical emotions in today's post-truth, digital age, scholarly attention to the relationship between suspicion and biomedical certainty offers due recognition to the affective workings of what Said-iya Hartman has famously called the "afterlife of slavery."[29] "If slavery persists as an issue," Hartman argues, "it is not because of an antiquarian obsession with bygone days or the burden of a too-long memory, but because black lives are still imperiled and devalued by a racial calculus and a political arithmetic that were entrenched centuries ago."[30] Thinking alongside transnational and women of color feminist theorizations of affect as I have in this book, the specifically em-bodied feelings, affective circuits, and interpretive frames through which Afro-Barbadians contextualize the Barbadian state's medicopharmaceutical biopol-itics are aptly engaged. By foregrounding the palimpsestic life of suspicion, I have outlined an epistemic argument about suspicion and its relationship to certainty, care, and protection for many Afro-Barbadian parents in postcolonial Barbados—one that need not conflict with on-the-ground public health efforts to improve vaccine compliance and prevent cervical cancer but in fact should urgently inform and enrich these energies and support the holistic health of our populations with an ethics of radical care.

CONCLUSION

Toward Radical Care

Throughout this book, I have been thinking of these questions: What logics and histories underlie understandings of vaccine hesitancy as irrational and conspiratorial? Of what significance is Afro-Barbadians' vernacular expression of hesitancy as suspicion? How is suspicion articulated, and to what ends? Where does suspicion circulate and with what effects? What does suspicion offer to Afro-Barbadians, to scholars, and to medical practitioners?

Beginning by situating the contemporary language of vaccine hesitancy and its preclusions in a lineage of medical discourse on noncompliance and nonadherence, I show how terms such as *hesitancy* participate in a culture of biomedicine that is often frustratingly inattentive to the weight history continues to bear on peoples of African descent as they encounter and navigate neoliberal policies, mushrooming state–industry partnerships, and their pharmaceutical and technological offerings. Unfaithful to biomedical understandings of vaccine hesitancy as the delay or complete refusal of vaccines in the context of available immunization services, I engaged with the stories and claims of middle-class Afro-Barbadian parents, Barbadian public health practitioners, and adolescents to whom the HPV vaccine is targeted to offer a theory of suspicion as an instinctual, vernacularized, and generative reframing of hesitancy.

Suspicion, I asserted, is the affective expression of emotions that Afro-Barbadians attach to the HPV vaccine, amid and alongside a range of burgeoning bio- and information technologies in twenty-first-century Barbados. Suspicion encapsulates but transcends hesitancy in the biomedical sense—more capaciously existing as an affective intensity and palimpsest of the long, racialized history of transatlantic slavery and its enmeshment in infrastructures of risk, capitalism, and biopolitical surveillance in Barbados and the anglophone Caribbean. Suspicion tells of Afro-Barbadians' embodied feelings of these colonial residues and engenders forms of skepticism through which they might unthinkably reason to protect their children by refusing medical technologies like the HPV vaccine and the processes of pharmaceuticalization in which it and the Barbadian state are impossibly enmeshed. Indeed, as I argue in chapter 1, beyond the scope of the HPV vaccine, suspicion exists more capaciously alongside and in response to Barbados's precarious economy and the state's shifting forms of neoliberal governmentality.

When I began this research in 2015, Barbados was just beginning to see glimmers of recovery after a six-year economic recession. Even so, societal concerns over job security, government accountability, and distrust toward intraregional migrants remained palpable. Throughout this book I traced how Afro-Barbadians' experiences of suspicion in relation to regional migrants and arrangements like the Caribbean Skilled Market Economy (CSME) circulate in the same economies as those surrounding technologies like the HPV vaccine. Punctuating their suspicions about the vaccine with criticisms of their government's facilitation of intraregional migration, concerns over foreign investments, and interests in Barbadian companies made possible through neoliberal configurations like the CSME, Afro-Barbadians in this book made clear the entanglement of suspicion with these socioeconomic and political moves that the state has undertaken since the late 2000s—of which the introduction of the HPV vaccine was just one. Contextualizing suspicion in these and longer histories, I framed the significance of economic uncertainty, state retreat, and a brooding sense of government distrust with reference to Afro-Barbadians' reception and deliberation of state initiatives such as (but not limited to) the HPV vaccination program introduced in 2014.

In this book I have made two overarching arguments. The first speaks to suspicion's effects for and implications on the Afro-Barbadian parents for whom it is a lived reality. Suspicion, I have shown, is a generative affective pedagogy that engenders feelings of protection and refusal for Afro-Barbadian parents. Suspicion holds the potential to shape not only their engagements with technologies like the HPV vaccine but their (dis)engagement with claims to certainty and knowledge about hesitancy, care, and protection made by various state and industry actors. As suspicion attaches to the capitalist interests behind the pharmaceutical promotion of the vaccine and historical tropes of hypersexuality and erotic subjugation under slavery, the term *hesitancy*'s "historical" tropes are revealed, exposing the persistence of histories of racialized science in the twenty-first century and Afro-Barbadians' warranted concerns of the same. As parents expressed, suspicion is prudent and protective from these injurious realities.

Yet as an affect that claims to provide protection, suspicion is simultaneously fallible. Like the precarious and unstable discourses of biomedical certainty espoused by Barbadian doctors and nurses, this book has made clear suspicion's fraught nature and inescapable shortcomings amid high rates of cervical cancer in the Caribbean. Should suspicion continue to result in forms of refusal and therefore low HPV vaccine uptake rates in Barbados, this will probably result in serious health implications, including disease and death, for the very teenagers whose parents are seeking protection via suspicion and vaccine refusal. Fraught as it is, this book highlights that suspicion ought not to be simply something to be overcome but instead understood for its gestures toward less injurious forms of health care promotion.

Another central argument of this book has been that suspicion is empirically significant. When we understand suspicion as affective, it necessarily complicates biomedical narratives around suspicion and hesitancy as merely fraught and irrational refusals of biomedical protection. Suspicious affects, I show, promise capacious insights for public health and medical practitioners and for transnational feminist, (techno)science, and humanities scholars alike, who might be hesitant to produce conceptually neat end points to inescapably entangled biopolitics of past and present. Put simply, suspicion interrogates the biomedical offerings of care presented via the HPV vaccine. In so doing, it reveals care's inequalities and political stakes by mapping how health care work, biomedical authority, state priorities, assemblages, and noninnocent histories of colonial medical injustice often unwittingly intertwine. I believe that failing to attend to these considerations diminishes the efficacy of public health efforts to improve vaccine compliance and can bring serious unintended consequences.

This book ultimately offers a call to think about suspicion as generative theory and praxis, and this call invites us to think about radical care. What if suspicion were staged as a generative form of radical care and collectivity? As I have argued for here, what if suspicion is recognized as an affective attachment that refuses discourses of irrationality and ignorance in favor of embodying a radical potential to teach of a care rooted in deep witnessing and reflection as a precursor to prescription, mediation, and medical innovations? Radical care, as I explained in chapter 4, is built on a set of collective sociopolitical and ethical considerations toward an otherwise.[1] Through the affective and corporeal sensation of suspicion, Afro-Barbadian parents herein demonstrate what it means to instrumentalize a collective capacity for radical care—a caring otherwise, outside colonial and scientific claims to objectivity and rationality, process of pharmaceuticalization, neoliberal governmentality, and state–industry partnerships, all through which the HPV vaccine comes to be realized. Following the generativity of suspicion in an effort to rethink care around HPV, cervical and other HPV-related cancers, and health effects in Barbados is thus to embrace the ambivalence of care, biomedical certainty, and the HPV vaccine. It is to compassionately recognize the powerful affective competence and residue of histories of community-engaged learning and capacity-building around Caribbean women's health, histories of bio- and necropolitics around and on the Black woman's body, and Barbados's neoimperial, neoliberal, and postcolonial contemporary. Overdrawing the opposition between suspicion and biomedical certainty in an attempt to overcome the former threatens to limit our attention to what these rubrics collectively offer scholars and health care practitioners seeking to understand the racialized, gendered, historical, and affective politics of care and its presumed impediments.

Coda

Five years since my first research trip to Barbados, I write this conclusion five months into the COVID-19 pandemic. The Barbadian prime minister's calls for increased regional integration to aid economic development throughout the region—especially in places like Suriname and Guyana, which have seen recent discoveries of significant offshore oil reserves—have been put on hold indefinitely. Although astronomical gains were projected for the CARICOM community in light of these oil discoveries, COVID's induced oil oversupply has changed these prospects overnight. In addition to the decline in tourism, the virus has left economists projecting a regional recession of an unpredictable duration alongside the inevitable global financial crisis and has amplified the post-independence struggle to create stable and diverse economies for citizens of the region.

Amid increasing precarity, suspicions linger. In April 2020, news broke that the United States had restricted the export of twenty ventilators that were donated to Barbados where most of the initial COVID-19 cases were, unsurprisingly, from tourists or from those who had been to the United States.[2] In newspaper commentaries, Barbadians were quick to criticize the Trump administration and its export ban. As with their critique of the pharmaceutical company Merck, they pointed to the extractive presence of foreign interests and countries in Barbados even and especially during a global pandemic when the Ministry of Health was seeking more health care workers to assist in the COVID-19 fight. By blocking Barbados and other countries from acquiring some of the most in-demand medical equipment, the United States highlights its capacity to engage in a "modern form of piracy" that effectively bars acts of philanthropy toward the small island nation, with significant humanitarian and socioeconomic implications.[3]

Farther away (perhaps only in geographical terms), two French doctors suggested that the COVID-19 vaccine be tested on the African continent. In April 2020, in reference to the trials set to begin in Europe and Australia using a BCG tuberculosis vaccine, Jean-Paul Mira, head of the Intensive Care Unit at Cochin Hospital in Paris, claimed: "If I could be provocative, should we not do this study in Africa where there are no masks, treatment or intensive care, a little bit like it's done, by the way, for certain AIDS studies or with prostitutes. . . . We try things because we know that they are highly exposed and they don't protect themselves."[4] Supporting Mira's egregious assertion, Camille Locht, research director of the French National Institute of Health and Medical Research (Inserm) noted, "You are right. And by the way, we are in the process of thinking in parallel about a study in Africa."[5] After international backlash and outrage on social media, Inserm defended Locht's racist suggestions by posting a tweet of their own beginning with the words "#FakeNews" that went on to suggest that Locht's comments were merely misinterpreted.[6]

The connections between these regional and international geopolitical events, the longue durée of colonial medical racism transnationally and their intersections with claims to fake news in a post-truth era, and the affects of suspicion described in this book cannot be overlooked. As many of the Afro-Barbadian parents expressed, suspicion toward the intent of biomedical intervention among Black populations is not without precedent. Indebted to a transnational feminist praxis which, as M. Jacqui Alexander and Chandra Mohanty note, is location specific but not bound, the theory of suspicion I have outlined herein implores us to attend to the past histories of transatlantic slavery and medical experimentation (which undoubtedly inhere in the present) in and beyond the Caribbean.[7] A transnational lens asks that we account for this history's ideological proximity to many of the ongoing transnational policies and socioeconomic forms of dispossession that affect peoples of the African diaspora today and that we refuse the impulse to immediately dismiss these unsettling continuities as fake or conspiratorial.

This book contributes to critical feminist technoscience studies of postcolonial biopolitics, the ambivalence of biomedicine, and a body of transnational Black feminist scholarship attuned to the afterlives of slavery; the movement and mobilization of power, relationality, and affect across space and time; and the exacerbated inequalities produced by neoliberalism in the anglophone Caribbean and beyond. I have emphasized the continued salience of histories of persistent colonialism-capitalism, of which science and medicine were and seem to remain an integral part. Suspicion, I have shown, disconcertingly exposes these realities.

Rethinking suspicion and care calls on medical practitioners and public health workers to release investments in conceiving hesitancy as a refusal of care, in conceiving suspicion and refusal as subsumed within scientific ignorance, and in conceiving vaccine acceptance as a value-neutral willingness to receive care. Furthermore, and more challenging, it requires that social science and scientific researchers/practitioners critically reflect on our conditioned means of studying and offering care; listen more closely to and wrestle with how biomedicine's rationalities around care intersect with histories of injustice, postcolonial state building, and contemporary neoliberal priorities and agendas; and accept the ways these rationalities might be understood to inflict more harm than good. Suspicion, suspicious refusals, ambivalence, and hesitancy hold up a mirror to the violence often implicit in our caring and naming practices. They unveil the histories of care and the lingering power of historical narratives of ignorance that surface in discourses of vaccine hesitancy and refusal. They necessitate that we pause to more ethically revisit the question of care.

Heeding Michel-Rolph Trouillot's call to shift the lens of analysis inward, to a small place, to capture the "agentive capacities of ordinary people" amid evolving and converging historical and contemporary processes of domination, this book has sought to map the not-so-obvious stakes of biomedical modes of care and suspicion toward that care in the context of postcolonial Barbados.[8] From this perspective, we are faced with care's underbelly. Indeed, as the Afro-Barbadian parents whom I interviewed have offered, when framed in a noninnocent history of biomedical experimentation and "care," (post)colonial stereotypes and politics, and pharmaceutical-state assemblages, the historical etymology of the word *care* and its conflation with fear, anxiety, and grief seems more intuitive.

In describing their suspicion, Afro-Barbadian parents collectively repositioned the crisis of cervical cancer in the Caribbean (indeed, the crisis of caring for this crisis) in and against the anxious paternalism of the postcolonial state and histories of surveillance and neglect, colonialism, biomedical experimentation, and suspicion toward Black women and Black women's (hyper)sexuality in Barbados and transnationally. In so doing, they complicate what it means to be suspicious of (the care of) this vaccine in a place like Barbados and amid popular understandings of vaccine hesitancy and refusal in the Western world. Eschewing the binaries that structure(d) colonial discourse and medical discourse around rationality and irrationality, suspicion implores us to look more closely at the enmeshment of risk, care, and fear in the postcolonial Caribbean.

Beyond the Caribbean and the HPV vaccine, this theoretical framing of suspicion and its gestures to radical care offers us a framework to think transnationally about the seemingly disparate interests in refusing the HPV vaccine in Barbados, testing COVID-19 vaccines on Black people within the African continent, attacks against Médecins sans frontières workers seeking to intervene in the Ebola epidemic in the Democratic Republic of Congo, and the US seizure of medical equipment destined for Barbados amid a global pandemic which gestures to futures of pernicious vaccine apartheid and nationalism in relation to COVID-19 vaccines.[9] Suspicion asks that social science and humanities researchers and health care practitioners alike recognize these as ideologically proximate and push us to recognize and accept the histories, genealogies, and practices of care that we might yet comprehend. To follow suspicion and rethink care is to embrace the ambivalence of care and biomedical technologies like vaccines and the incomprehensible, seemingly impossible not-doing that hesitancy might constitute in favor of compassionate recognition, close listening, reflection, and cautious pause. And perhaps this is radical.

Notes

Portions of this introduction appeared in "HPV Vaccination and Affective Suspicions in Barbados," *Feminist Formations* 30, no. 1 (Spring 2018): 46–70.

1. Reddit, "Make This Skeptical Kid into a Meme, STAT!"
2. CDC, "HPV Vaccine Prevents HPV."
3. CDC, "HPV Vaccine Prevents HPV."
4. HPV Information Centre, "Human Papillomavirus and Related Diseases."
5. HPV Information Centre, "Human Papillomavirus and Related Diseases."
6. See Durbach, *Bodily Matters*; Conis, *Vaccine Nation*.
7. Council of Foreign Relations, "Map: Vaccine-Preventable Outbreaks."
8. WHO, "Vaccine Hesitancy."
9. WHO, "Report of the SAGE Working Group."
10. WHO, "Report of the SAGE Working Group."
11. WHO, "Report of the SAGE Working Group."
12. Larson et al., "Addressing the Vaccine Confidence Gap"; Naus, "What Do We Know about How to Improve Vaccine Uptake?"; WHO, "Report of the SAGE Working Group."
13. Poltorak et al., "'MMR Talk' and Vaccination Choices"; Leach and Fairhead, *Vaccine Anxieties*; Goldenberg, "Public Misunderstanding of Science?"; Lawrence, Hausman, and Dannenberg, "Reframing Medicine's Publics."
14. See Closser et al., "Global Context of Vaccine Refusal"; Ghinai et al., "Listening to the Rumours."
15. See Offit, *Deadly Choices* and "Junk Science Isn't a Victimless Crime."
16. The terms *Afro-Barbadian* or *Afro-Bajan* are used interchangeably throughout this book to refer to Barbadians who are of entirely or predominantly African descent.
17. Greene, "Therapeutic Infidelities," 329.
18. See Trostle, "Medical Compliance as an Ideology"; Greene, "Therapeutic Infidelities"; Keller, "Geographies of Power."

19. For instance, see Biehl, "Pharmaceuticalization"; Das and Das, "Pharmaceuticals in Urban Ecologies"; Maskovsky, "Do People Fail Drugs?"; Whitmarsh, "Medical Schismogenics."

20. Whitmarsh, "Medical Schismogenics."

21. WHO, "Report of the SAGE Working Group." The term *vaccine hesitancy* emerged following a WHO November 2011 meeting of the Strategic Advisory Group of Experts (SAGE) on immunization and the establishment of a working group dedicated specifically to dealing with the problem of hesitancy and its effect on vaccination uptake rates. According to my PubMed and Scopus searches, the phrase *vaccine hesitancy* relatedly began to appear prominently in medical literature from 2011, largely replacing the use of the terms *acceptance* and *compliance*.

22. See King, *Black Shoals*; Tinsley, "Black Atlantic, Queer Atlantic"; Sharpe, *In the Wake*; R. Walcott, *Black Like Who?*

23. See Morgensen, *Spaces between Us*; Tuck and Yang, "Decolonization Is Not a Metaphor"; Snelgrove, Dhamoon, and Corntassel, "Unsettling Settler Colonialism."

24. See Murphy, "Unsettling Care"; Philip, "Keep on Copyin' in the Free World"; Haraway, *Staying with the Trouble*.

25. The Global Alliance for Vaccines and Immunization is an international alliance of public health and nonprofit partners that has been instrumental in improving access to immunization services in the developing world, lobbying for cost-effective vaccines, and advocating for the research and development of vaccines therein.

26. For a discussion on Black feminist conceptions of the visual practice/tactic of and commitment to refusal, see Campt, "Black Visuality and the Practice of Refusal."

27. As many feminist and postcolonial scholars have highlighted, the term *postcolonial* itself reproduces a binary of time, such that it suggests that historical events are not currently involved in the present. See McClintock, *Imperial Leather*; Shohat, "Notes on the 'Post-Colonial.'" I use the term *postcolonial* throughout this book simply to designate the time period after which Barbados achieved independence from Britain, cognizant of the term's problematic linguistic emphasis on the colonial narrative and in appreciation and recognition of the multiplicities of space, place, and time that inhere in the contemporary.

28. World Bank, "Population, Total: Data."

29. See DaCosta, *Colonial Origins, Institutions and Economic Performance*.

30. US Central Intelligence Agency, "World Factbook: Barbados Economy."

31. Charles-Soverall and Khan, "Social Partnership," 22–24. Included in this social partnership agreement with the government were industries and businesses, trade unions, and community and participant organizations, all of which agreed to work together to develop strategies to manage the economy and build strong institutions that would resist economic threats.

32. Falling international oil prices and a rebound in tourist arrivals in late 2015 began to improve the country's external economic position. Despite this, sociopolitical instability, unemployment, and public sector layoffs persisted among citizens during my first research trip to Barbados from 2015 to 2016.

33. In the May 2018 Barbadian general election, the BLP won with a landslide victory,

and BLP leader Mia Mottley became the country's first female prime minister. Mottley inherited a large national debt, which more than doubled over the DLP's ten-year reign, and quickly called in the assistance of the International Monetary Fund, suspended liability payments, and announced a three-phase five-year package of austerity measures to address the dire state of the economy.

34. The term *biocitizenship* has variously referred to the mobilization of citizens around their biological bodies as a resource for state recognition and support; citizenship projects and modes of self-formation in which persons use biological language to express their concerns, needs, rights, and entitlements; and the positive thinking about and improvement on one's biology through biotechnologies, patient activism, and other forms of political organizing. See Petryna, *Life Exposed*, 18; Rose and Novas, "Biological Citizenship"; Rose, *Politics of Life Itself*, 132–34. As I have critically argued elsewhere, biocitizenship also includes "the use of biological preconditions, or pre-damaged bodies, as a mobilizing force by the state and other authoritative channels, to recruit individuals . . . as bioconsumers and active biocitizens"; Charles, "Mobilizing the Self-Governance," 780. Although biocitizenship might offer citizens hope in science and medicine for enabling cures and treatment for biological maladies, these "new biotechnologies now also . . . demand the responsibility and duty to seek care and cures" in ways that are "largely capitalist and neoliberal and neglect issues of social location"; Charles, "Mobilizing the Self-Governance," 772. For further Black feminist and technoscience critiques of biocitizenship scholarship and its overwhelming alignment with and emphasis on individual health and health consumption and neoliberal social and political logics, see Roberts, "Social Immorality of Health," 61; Benjamin, *People's Science*, 17.

35. Charles, "Mobilizing the Self-Governance," 776.

36. As of 2016, several other Caribbean countries have also implemented national HPV vaccination programs, including Anguilla, Bahamas, Barbados, Bermuda, Cayman Islands, Guyana, Suriname, and Trinidad and Tobago. See Hutton, "Mobilizing Civil Society." In 2017 Jamaica began offering the vaccine to girls through high schools. Saunders, "HPV Vaccine Administered."

37. In 2009, pharmaceutical company GlaxoSmithKline's vaccine Cervarix was approved by the FDA and indicated for use in girls and women between ten and twenty-five years to protect against the two types of HPV (16 and 18) that cause approximately 70 percent of all cervical cancer cases. Both Gardasil and Cervarix have since been discontinued in the United States in favor of Merck's latest HPV vaccine, Gardasil 9, which was approved in 2014 to treat nine HPV types (6, 11, 16, 18, 31, 33, 45, 52, and 58) that can variously lead to genital warts in women and men; cervical, vaginal, and vulvar cancers in women; anal and throat cancer in women and men; and penile cancer in men. During my fieldwork in Barbados, the quadrivalent vaccine was still being used as part of the national vaccination program.

38. Abbott, "Pharmaceutical Benefits Scheme." Australia was the first country to introduce a National HPV Vaccination Program for men in 2013, though it first began offering the vaccine in 2007 for women. Similarly, though Health Canada approved the use of the HPV vaccine for use in both girls and boys in 2010, it was not until 2013 that

the provinces of Prince Edward Island and Alberta announced their intention to extend their HPV vaccination programs to school-age boys. See CBC News, "P.E.I. Is Expanding." Several other Canadian provinces have since followed.

39. According to a senior medical officer at the Barbados Ministry of Health with whom I spoke, the initial decision to deliver the vaccine to preteen girls at school was modeled after international research and consultation which suggested it as an effective method both to target adolescents before they become sexually active and to ensure the multidose completion of the vaccine. The Global Vaccine Alliance indicates that school-based delivery has resulted in coverage rates of more than 80 percent in countries that piloted this method in HPV vaccine demonstration programs.

40. Personal communication, senior medical officer at the Barbadian Ministry of Health, October 2015.

41. Seymour, "Resistance"; Abu-Lughod, "Romance of Resistance."

42. See McGranahan, "Theorizing Refusal"; Redfield, "Doctors, Borders, and Life in Crisis"; Rapp, *Testing Women, Testing the Fetus*; Sobo, "Theorizing (Vaccine) Refusal"; Benjamin, "Informed Refusal."

43. Campt, "Black Visuality and the Practice of Refusal," 80.

44. Simpson, *Mohawk Interruptus*, 104–5.

45. TallBear, *Native American DNA*, 25.

46. Benjamin, *People's Science*, 153.

47. Benjamin, *People's Science*, 139.

48. For a capacious reading of affect across psychoanalytic, feminist, and philosophical traditions, see Gregg and Seigworth, *Affect Theory Reader*; Massumi, *Parables for the Virtual*; Sedgwick and Frank, *Touching Feeling*; Gorton, "Theorizing Emotion and Affect"; Ahmed, "Affective Economies"; Cvetkovich, *Archive of Feelings*.

49. Ahmed, "Affective Economies," 119. Teresa Brennan similarly invokes affect as sticky, contagious intensities. Arguing against the belief that affects are self-contained, Brennan adopts insights from neurology and biochemistry to illustrate how porous systems, atmospheres, and environments circulate and transfer in ways that quite literally "ge[t] into" individuals; Brennan, *Transmission of Affect*, 1. Although Brennan argues for this model of contagion via proximity, she makes clear the unequal ways affects are received and registered by individuals. Ahmed reiterates that affect does not merely transfer or "stick" between proximate bodies, but instead moves according to the inherent political and economic dimensions that undergird this stickiness; Ahmed, *Promise of Happiness*, 44.

50. See also Saldanha, "Political Geography of Many Bodies."

51. Patricia Clough describes the "turn to affect" as the scholarly move away from text, epistemology, and discourse and toward the materiality of reality that occurred during the early to mid-1990s; Clough, "Affective Turn," 1–2. See Hochschild, "Emotion Work"; Jaggar, "Love and Knowledge"; and Lorde, *Sister Outsider*, for examples of feminist scholarship that precede this "turn."

52. Lorde, *Uses of the Erotic*; Moraga, "Catching Fire," xix.

53. Garcia-Rojas, "(Un)Disciplined Futures," 3.

54. Garcia-Rojas, "(Un)Disciplined Futures."

55. Transnational feminist frameworks presuppose that critical knowledge about social and cultural processes is most effectively generated by foregrounding questions of race, sexuality, conquest, colonialism, and global capitalism. Theorists in this lineage are further attentive to how power is made and mediated across time and place and in socioeconomic and political structures, systemic laws, governmental policies, institutions, forms of media, and storytelling. See Alexander, *Pedagogies of Crossing*; Alexander and Mohanty, "Cartographies of Knowledge and Power"; Grewal and Kaplan, "Postcolonial Studies" and *Scattered Hegemonies*.

56. Alexander, *Pedagogies of Crossing*, 190. Here, Alexander draws on the work of cultural and feminist theorists invested in critiquing the dualism of time to forward this understanding of the palimpsest. See Grossberg, "History, Politics and Postmodernism"; Shohat, *Talking Visions*.

57. Alexander, *Pedagogies of Crossing*, 190.

58. Hall, "Local and the Global," 20.

59. See DeBarros, *Reproducing the British Caribbean*; Levine, *Prostitution, Race, and Politics*.

60. Alexander, *Pedagogies of Crossing*.

61. See Alexander, *Pedagogies of Crossing*; Alexander and Mohanty, "Cartographies of Knowledge and Power"; Grewal and Kaplan, *Scattered Hegemonies*.

62. In addition to a large body of Caribbean transnational feminist scholarship, see Alexander, "Not Just (Any)Body" and *Pedagogies of Crossing*; Sheller, *Citizenship from Below*; Trotz, "Rethinking Caribbean Transnational Connections." Scholars have similarly traced the transnational effects of contemporary experiences of neoliberal globalization on identity formation, diasporic modes of resistance and expression, and forms of labor across the African diaspora. See King, *Black Shoals*; Philip, *Caribana*; Tinsley, "Black Atlantic, Queer Atlantic"; Tinsley et al., "So Much to Remind Us."

63. See Alexander, *Pedagogies of Crossing*; Puri, *Caribbean Postcolonial*; Sheller, *Citizenship from Below*; Thomas, *Exceptional Violence*.

64. My sample of interview participants consisted of twenty-eight parents and legal guardians, all of whom self-identified as middle-class and were between the ages of thirty-one and fifty-one years. Of these parents, twenty-four identified as Black, three as white, and one as mixed race. They encompassed individuals from each of Barbados's eleven parishes or subregions, with most concentrated in the parishes of St. James, Christ Church, and St. Michael, the latter of which is home to the nation's capital of Bridgetown. I interviewed a total of eighteen medical professionals, including senior medical officers at the Barbadian Ministry of Health, private pediatricians, general practitioners, obstetricians, and gynecologists as well as immunization nurses throughout the nine publicly funded polyclinics that were responsible for distributing the HPV vaccine through the national program. Seventeen of these practitioners identified as Black, and one as Indian-Caribbean. I interviewed fourteen teenagers ranging in age from fourteen to nineteen years, twelve of whom self-identified as Black or Afro-Caribbean, one as Indian-Caribbean, and one as white. To protect participants' privacy, pseudonyms are used, with the exception of the names of public figures which appeared in local newspapers, online, or on social media.

65. "Bajan" is a commonly used local term to refer to a Barbadian. I use the terms interchangeably throughout this book.

66. As I explain in chapter 1, this suspicion around my status and the aims of my research can be understood in the wider context of Barbadians' underlying skepticism of the motives of international pharmaceutical companies and clinical trial organizations, which have become increasingly interested in recruiting Barbadians as participants in drug research trials on diseases from cancer and asthma to heart disease and diabetes. See Whitmarsh, *Biomedical Ambiguity*. Interestingly, though, for some participants, my affiliation with the University of Toronto was positively received. I suspect this disparity is because my Canadian background at times overshadowed my Trinidadian identity. On more than one occasion, participants referred to Trinidadians as "Trickidadians," meaning vindictive or deceitful—specifically in the context of purchasing and profiting off Barbadian businesses and property.

67. The parents I interviewed collectively resided across all of Barbados's eleven parishes, which enabled me to capture an understanding of the similarities between parents' concerns across the island. Twenty of these parents identified as "HPV vaccine hesitant" and either previously declined the HPV vaccination for their children or had intentions of refusing the vaccine in the near future. Two described themselves as undecided yet "suspicious." Three of the parents I interviewed accepted the vaccine for their children but were eager to share their stories with me either because of a lingering uncertainty or ambivalence about their decision, an unfavorable experience with the vaccine, or to describe their emphatic views about the cultural taboos they believed were driving resistance to the vaccine.

68. All Barbadian girls and boys of the target age group can receive the vaccine free of charge through the public clinics. As such, it was common for the parents I interviewed to accompany their children to receive the vaccine at the polyclinic that correlated with the subregion where they lived or where their children attended school. In my conversation with a local pediatrician, he noted that the vaccine had recently become available through private practitioners, but because of its high cost, it was almost exclusively being administered to those who were ineligible to receive it through the Ministry of Health.

69. Hartman, *Lose Your Mother*, 6.

CHAPTER ONE. CIRCLES OF SUSPICION

Sections of this chapter appeared in "HPV Vaccination and Affective Suspicions in Barbados," *Feminist Formations* 30, no. 1 (Spring 2018): 46–70.

1. Republic Bank Limited, "Subsidiaries."

2. Immunization Nurse Dobbs, interview with author, October 2015. Direct quotes for all interview excerpts are kept in the original form, which includes Barbadian dialect and standardized English.

3. Ahmed, *Promise of Happiness*, 24.

4. WHO, "Vaccine Hesitancy."

5. Alexander, *Pedagogies of Crossing*, 190.

6. Ifill, "Transformation of the Sphere of Governance."

7. Caribbean Community (CARICOM) Secretariat, "Revised Treaty." The treaty establishing CARICOM, the Treaty of Chaguaramas, originally drafted in 1973, first provided for the creation of two distinct entities: the Caribbean Community and the Common Market. With the proposal of CSME, CARICOM hoped to create a more unified market space than under the former treaty, one in which the development and production of services, goods, and labor could be integrated into the global economy.

8. While CARICOM comprises fourteen Caribbean countries, only twelve have fully signed on to participate in the free movement of CARICOM nationals under the CSME. These countries include Barbados, Antigua and Barbuda, Belize, Dominica, Grenada, Guyana, Jamaica, St. Kitts and Nevis, St. Lucia, St. Vincent and the Grenadines, Suriname, and Trinidad and Tobago. For more on CARICOM, see Brathwaite, "CARICOM and the Politics of Migration."

9. Arthur, "Address."

10. World Bank, "World Development Indicators."

11. See United Nations Development Programme, "Human Development Reports, 2018." The Human Development Index is a composite measure of three aspects of development: education, health, and income.

12. Newstead, "Regional Governmentality."

13. For a nuanced analysis of the varying effects of globalization on racial relations, cultural production, and economic change in anglophone Caribbean societies, see Brereton, "All Ah We Is Not One"; Thomas and Clarke, *Globalization and Race*; Murray, *Flaming Souls*.

14. Freeman, *Entrepreneurial Selves*.

15. Arthur, "Address."

16. Arthur, "Address."

17. For more on fears around cross-border politics in Barbados around the CSME, see Brathwaite, "CARICOM and the Politics of Migration." See Girvan, "'Real' Immigration Problem," which details the effects Guyanese, Vincentian, and St. Lucian workers have held on the Barbadian economy in the early years of the CSME's implementation.

18. Brathwaite, "CARICOM and the Politics of Migration."

19. Wickham et al., "Freedom of Movement," 53.

20. Wickham et al., "Freedom of Movement," 53.

21. Caribbean Court of Justice, "'Caribbean Court of Justice."

22. Artaxerxes, comment on David, "Hegemony of Trinidad."

23. Bush Tea, comment on David, "Hegemony of Trinidad."

24. Ministry of Labour and Immigration, "Comprehensive Review of Immigration Policy."

25. Brathwaite, "CARICOM and the Politics of Migration."

26. Brandford, "PM's Case for Fingerprinting."

27. Brandford, "PM's Case for Fingerprinting."

28. Murray, *Flaming Souls*, 6.

29. For more on bioavailable zones and biomedicalization, see Clarke et al., "Biomedicalization," 9. Ian Whitmarsh discusses Barbados's appeal as an international center

of genetics-of-disease research premised on race as a result of multiple factors, including the country's "nationalized health care system and integration into global medical markets," a racially homogeneous population of Afro-Caribbean people, and a highly educated and literate populace that is perceived to value medical care and thus be more amenable to research participation. Whitmarsh, *Biomedical Ambiguity*, 34.

30. Whitmarsh, *Biomedical Ambiguity*.

31. Many Barbadian public health professionals use the pseudonyms John Public and John Q. Public to refer to lay citizens and members of the general public.

32. Antrobus, "Entrepreneurial Selves."

33. Antrobus, "Entrepreneurial Selves," 562.

34. Freeman, *Entrepreneurial Selves*, 214.

CHAPTER TWO. RISK AND SUSPICION

An earlier version of chapter 2 appeared in "Suspicion and/as Radical (Care): Looking Closer at Vaccine Hesitancy in Postcolonial Barbados," *Social Text* 38, no. 1 (142): 89–107.

1. Beck, *Risk Society*.

2. Beck, "Terrorist Threat," 40–41.

3. Levy, *Freaks of Fortune*.

4. Levy, *Freaks of Fortune*, 3.

5. See Levy, *Freaks of Fortune*; Schlich, "Risk and Medical Innovation."

6. See Schlich, "Risk and Medical Innovation"; Magnello, "Introduction of Mathematical Statistics"; Zachmann, "Risk in Historical Perspective."

7. See Schlich, "Risk and Medical Innovation."

8. See Schlich, "Risk and Medical Innovation"; Marks, "Assessing the Risk and Safety of the Pill"; Rusnock, "'Merchant's Logick.'"

9. Brown, *Immunitary Life*, 175.

10. See Altink, "'Fight TB with BCG.'" As Altink notes, while BCG vaccination campaigns against tuberculosis in the mid-twentieth-century British Caribbean were promoted through the lens of public health and its benefits for political, social, and economic advancement, such initiatives ultimately aimed to reinvigorate the British empire.

11. Bonah, "As Safe as Milk or Sugar Water.'"

12. Foucault, *History of Sexuality*.

13. Schlich, "Risk and Medical Innovation," 5.

14. See Casper and Carpenter, "Sex, Drugs, and Politics." See also Connell and Hunt, "HPV Vaccination Campaign"; Lock and Nguyen, "Biomedical Technologies in Practice."

15. Sagicor Life, "Sagicor and the Barbados Cancer Society."

16. Sagicor Life is a highly successful financial services company established in Barbados in 1840 as a life insurance company. Today, Sagicor provides a range of financial services, including life and health insurance, residential and commercial mortgages, pension investment, mutual funds, and asset management.

17. The other is the hepatitis B virus vaccine, which prevents a common form of liver cancer. See Mamo and Epstein, "Pharmaceuticalization of Sexual Risk."

18. Biocapitalism indicates an important shift in the constitution of symptoms to be treated and cared for "away from disease manifestation and toward disease potential"; Sunder Rajan, *Biocapital*, 283. Such a shift necessarily expands the potential market for pharmaceuticals "from 'diseased' people to conceivably everyone with purchasing power"; Sunder Rajan, "Subjects of Speculation," 24. The excessive biocapitalist influence of the pharmaceutical industry in Barbados does not go unnoticed by Barbadian health care practitioners and citizens.

19. Here risk attaches discursively almost exclusively to adolescent girls, their reproductive systems, and their sexuality despite the vaccine's administration through government-funded polyclinics to Barbadian girls and boys, who can also transmit HPV and develop genital warts and forms of cancer through persistent infection with the virus. As chapter 3 outlines, like the marketing of the vaccine, parents' concerns about the risks of HPV and of the vaccine are distinctly gendered.

20. Cordel et al., "High-Risk Human Papillomavirus"

21. Ward et al., "Human Papillomavirus Genotype Distribution."

22. Sheller, *Citizenship from Below*, 249.

23. De Barros, *Reproducing the British Caribbean*, 35. In the wake of widespread cholera epidemics in the 1850s and resulting labor shortages in such places as Barbados, Jamaica, and Trinidad, a medical tax system was imposed in many islands. British physicians reasoned that by taxing populations to pay for medical care, they could maintain dominance and economic profit in the colonies and train Black people on the benefits of rational, scientific advice in lieu of irrational, folk, and obeah quackery prescriptions.

24. Browne, *Race, Class, Politics.*

25. See Paton, "Enslaved Women and Slavery"; Challenger, "Benign Place of Healing?"; De Barros, *Reproducing the British Caribbean*; Putnam, "Global Child-Saving"; Bourbonnais, "Out of the Boudoir."

26. See Paton, "Enslaved Women and Slavery." Prior to 1780s, there was little interest in optimizing enslaved women's reproduction, but by the 1790s, planters and colonial officials became increasingly suspicious of enslaved women's attempts to abort or delay childbearing and began a fervent effort to maximize their labor supply by increasing imports and implementing pronatalist policies across Barbados, Jamaica, and the Leeward Islands to ensure a natural increase in laborers. Thus, interest in promoting biopolitical measures to optimize women's reproduction largely emerged in the late eighteenth century as abolition approached. Entries from Englishman Thomas Thistlewood's diary in the late 1760s offer insight into the routine violence and brutal sexual assault imposed on enslaved men and women across the English Caribbean before abolition. Thistlewood served as an estate manager in Jamaica, and he details the coercive necropolitical measures imposed on rebellious enslaved women, some of whom were pregnant, including flogging, the use of iron collars to chain women together by the necks, shackles, and the pickling of the wounded flesh of the enslaved with lime and pepper. See Delle, *Colonial Caribbean.*

27. Beckles, "Capitalism, Slavery, and Caribbean Modernity."

28. Paugh, *Politics of Reproduction*, 236.

29. Biopolitical incentives to replace imported Africans with Afro-Caribbean laborers were fundamentally schemes to "remoul[d] Afro-Caribbean sexuality and promot[e] Afro-Caribbean fertility"; Paugh, "Politics of Childbearing," 159.

30. See Beckles, *History of Barbados*. According to Beckles, at the turn of the nineteenth century, in addition to the medical and scientific surveillance of Black women's bodies, the rationale of "science" was increasingly drawn on by colonial officials across the British Caribbean to forward the notion of innate biological differences between Black and white people so that Black subjects were constructed as dangerous, premodern, irrational beings who lacked intelligence. The expansion of slums in Bridgetown, Barbados, and the spread of diseases like yellow fever, dysentery, smallpox, and measles throughout the British Caribbean in first half the nineteenth century only fueled these racialized beliefs that Blacks were uncivilized and incapable of preventing the spread of disease. For colonial planters and British officials, such epidemics and unsanitary living conditions symbolized the unpreparedness of former enslaved people to become respectable, health-conscious, and sanitary citizens. In Barbados, Beckles notes a government disinterest in implementing disease-preventative measures and improving the health conditions of Black people, except for quarantine measures that separated poor, unemployed, and diseased populations in generally unsuccessful attempts to control the spread of disease to colonial planters. For instance, in the wake of widespread cholera epidemics in the 1850s in places like Barbados, Jamaica, and Trinidad, which led to serious labor shortages, white planters (influenced by Victorian ideals and racial attitudes of Blacks as uncivilized, lazy, and barbarous) decried the spread of cholera as reflective of the moral failings of the formerly enslaved. "Civilized" white physicians and their biomedical tools were deemed the only remedy to counter the risks that poverty and Blackness were framed to pose. According to Juanita De Barros, during this period, British doctors were dispatched to the region and recommended a series of sanitary measures, which they soon determined were ineffective in addressing the poverty, climate, and geography that were further contributors to the spread of cholera. A subsequent medical tax system was imposed in many islands to "encourage the population to work" and discourage "idleness and savage[ry]"; De Barros, *Reproducing the British Caribbean*, 35.

31. De Barros, *Reproducing the British Caribbean*.

32. Leonard P. Fletcher, "Evolution of Poor Relief in Barbados, 1838–1900," *Journal of Caribbean History* 26, no. 2 (1992): 173, quoted in Green, "The 1938–1939 Moyne Commission," 520.

33. De Barros, *Reproducing the British Caribbean*.

34. LaFont, "Very Straight Sex."

35. See Gilman, "Black Bodies, White Bodies." Gilman notes how these racialized discourses of uncontrolled and immoral Black sexuality developed in the nineteenth century, bolstered by exhibitions such as those of the Hottentot woman. Along with other Black women brought from South Africa, Sartjie (Sarah) Baartman, who came to be known as the Hottentot Venus, was objectified for her "primitive" genitalia and buttocks and thus was labeled more sexually inclined and "intensive"; Gilman, "Black

Bodies, White Bodies," 212. These displays reinforced not only emergent medico-scientific constructions, but also how "the public display of Sartjee's lone, naked body, abstracted from familial or domestic context, underscored black women's exclusion from the prevailing cult of domesticity"; Jones, "Human Weeds, Not Fit to Breed?," 51. Thus, apart from sexualizing and racializing Blackness, narratives of hypersexuality spatially confined and restricted the mobility of Black women transnationally from the nineteenth century. In the anglophone Caribbean, these discourses functioned in similar ways to criminalize Blackness and further naturalize whiteness. While Black women's bodies were formulated as unruly and bestial and Black men as threatening and hypersexual, whiteness and its standards of piety and morality were crystallized as ideals to be upheld. See Alexander, "Not Just (Any) Body." By the twentieth century, it is no surprise that these pathologized discourses of the untamed, hyperfecund Black subject continued to underscore imperialist constructs of Blackness and the spread of venereal diseases. The proliferation of these eugenicist "scientific" beliefs rationalized Black women's violent abuses, including sexual exploitation and lynching, and subjected them to seemingly benevolent biopolitical medical interventions and experimentations that were in fact rooted in colonial anxieties about the Black body as a form of racial poison. See Levine, *Prostitution, Race, and Politics.*

36. Challenger, "Benign Place of Healing?" Contagious diseases laws were passed throughout the British Caribbean, first in Jamaica in 1867, followed by Barbados in 1868 and Trinidad in 1869. Unlike in Britain and in other British colonies, however, these laws extended to Barbados's civilian population, making any woman suspected of sex work subject to policing, invasive scrutiny, and "care."

37. Challenger, "Benign Place of Healing?"

38. Challenger, "Benign Place of Healing?," 106–7.

39. This historical degradation of Black women on account of their race, perceived lasciviousness, and view as racial poison could also be seen beyond the British empire in the United States. In response to these persistently degrading stereotypes, Black middle-class American women from the late nineteenth to the early twentieth century began to create new self-images and reconstruct the conception of Black female sexuality and immorality through politics of respectability and silence. See Higginbotham, *Righteous Discontent,* for a detailed discussion on the politics of respectability; Hine, "Rape and the Inner Lives." Politics of respectability eventually became indigenous to the formation of Black middle-class aspirations in America and the advancement of full citizenship for all Black Americans, and, as I discuss in this chapter, similarly manifested in Black middle-class nationalist discourses in the Caribbean in the 1960s. Notwithstanding new scientific and medical ideas about disease causation that continued to emerge during this period, suspicions about Black people's unsanitary living conditions were continually blamed for the transmission of communicable diseases and their sexual debauchery decried as responsible for the spread of venereal diseases and their associated social, political, and economic consequences through the 1920s.

40. Prompted by meager wages and labor conditions and white planters' apathetic approach to their health and social and living environments, working-class Barbadians began mobilizing. Inspired by pan-Africanism, Marxism, and Black nationalist Garvey-

ism (to name just a few radical traditions and philosophies), working-class citizens rallied against labor standards, social and living conditions, and overarching racial injustice and discrimination. By 1937, the decade-long political activism of the working class had planted the seeds for the warm reception of Trinidadian-born trade union leader Clement Payne. Payne arrived in Barbados to organize workers against racial discrimination and exploitation, attracting thousands to his meetings, in which he spoke out against the poverty and abject labor conditions Black people had been subjected to in Barbados and throughout the Caribbean. His powerful words roused restlessness among Afro-Barbadians, plagued with the plethora of social, economic, and health problems and the racist attitudes and indifference of merchant-planter elite. The spark for the country's infamous and deadly uprisings occurred after Payne was arrested and secretly deported to Trinidad in July 1937, inciting rioting and looting that left fourteen dead, many wounded, and hundreds imprisoned. These riots prompted a series of disturbances across the Caribbean, each an attempt to put an end to widespread socioeconomic injustice, "wage slavery," and a dependency rooted in colonialism; Lewis, "The Contestation of Race in Barbadian Society," 155. In Barbados and throughout the British Caribbean, these riots signaled Black resistance against widespread racism, injustice treatment, neglect, and violence from both plantation and colonial masters and members of the white middle class. For more on these labor riots, see Beckles, *History of Barbados*; Bolland, *Politics of Labour*; Chamberlain, *Empire and Nation-Building*.

41. See Green, "1938–1939 Moyne Commission"; Parker, *Brother's Keeper*; Putnam, "Global Child-Saving."

42. "West India Royal Commission Report," London (1945), 220, quoted in Edmonds and Girvan, "Child Care and Family Services," 229.

43. Putnam, "Global Child-Saving," 238.

44. Putnam, "Global Child-Saving."

45. Bourbonnais, "Out of the Boudoir."

46. Nicole Bourbonnais argues that in addition to advocating for birth control, some conservative elites from the 1930s to the 1960s further expressed interest in compulsory sterilization of the unfit, warning of the severe problems that would ensue "if the less energetic, and the less progressive sections of the people were to swarm the limits of their ability'"; de Lisser, "Editorial," *Gleaner*, 4 November 1929, 12, as cited in Bourbonnais, "Class, Colour and Contraception," 10. These sentiments echo those simultaneously occurring in islands like Puerto Rico, where efforts were underway to curb the fecundity of "relentlessly fertile," "demon mothers" through processes like sterilizations, injections of high doses of hormones, and often covert measures such as placing contraceptive agents in the water supply; Briggs, *Reproducing Empire*, 110. As in the British Caribbean, race and sexuality lay at the heart of US imperial beliefs about development, modernization, and self-governance. But beyond these similarly racially motivated anxieties and eugenic concerns that undergirded the support of birth control from white elites, Barbadian middle-class Black politicians, professionals, and reformist elites also advocated for birth control.

47. See Stycos and Back, *Control of Human Fertility*; Blake, *Family Structure in Jamaica*.

48. Bourbonnais, "Out of the Boudoir," 29.

49. Rowley, *Feminist Advocacy*.

50. For more on the BFPA, see Slavin and Bilsborrow, "Barbados Family Planning Association"; Massiah, "Population of Barbados"; Segal, *Population Policies in the Caribbean*. Shortly after the BFPA's establishment, Jamaica and Trinidad and Tobago developed their own national programs to support the distribution of birth control, which were built on voluntary bodies and international organizations like the International Planned Parenthood Federation. In contrast to the population strategies in places like Cuba that sought to reorganize and structurally change economic and social facets of life to reduce fertility, these programs relied on the persuasive tactics of volunteers to gently "convince couples of the wisdom of birth limitation" and on the benefit of medical technologies such as the Pill and intrauterine devices from the early 1950s and throughout the 1960s; Cross, *Urbanization and Urban Growth*, 67. Despite its overall success in reducing birth rates, these persuasion-based biopolitical measures were met with various forms of suspicion and opposition throughout the Caribbean. Most notably, many religious leaders opposed the government support and widespread distribution of birth control, arguing that it would spread immorality. See Bourbonnais, "Out of the Boudoir."

51. Massiah, "Population of Barbados."

52. Higginbotham, *Righteous Discontent*. Higginbotham describes a politics of respectability as self-imposed protective frameworks of secrecy and silence, which middle-class Black women in the United States adhered to by modeling Victorian values of modesty, respectability, and morality in the hopes of counteracting racist and discriminatory colonial narratives of their hypersexuality, maternal ignorance, and dangerous immorality. Beginning with missionaries and teachers in the Black Baptist Church, Black women promoted Victorian manners and morals among themselves and encouraged poor working-class Black women to follow suit by transforming and abandoning their behaviors, philosophies, and modes of expression, from folk culture to Sunday baseball. While Black church leaders rallied around Black communities and were successful in helping many to establish Black-owned businesses, a preoccupation with respectability and denouncement of Black modes of expression and ways of life simultaneously fostered class tensions between Black people. Higginbotham notes, "The Baptist women never conceded that rejection of white middle-class values by poor blacks afforded survival strategies, in fact spaces of resistance, albeit different from their own"; Higginbotham, *Righteous Discontent*, 150. By the mid-twentieth century, these politics of respectability became indigenous to the formation of Black middle-class aspirations in America, and the advancement of full citizenship for Black women and men. Across the British empire, national projects of the twentieth century similarly deployed ideologies of bourgeois respectability, patriarchal gender roles, and Victorian ideals of women's domesticity as the yardstick of civility and citizenship, with the middle classes in turn seeking socialization into the idealized norms of respectability. Reverberations of this politics of respectability could be seen in the British Caribbean, coinciding with the rise of nationalism in the 1960s. See Alexander, "Redrafting Morality" and "Not Just (Any) Body"; Morris, *Close Kin and Distant Relatives*; Sheller, *Citi-*

zenship from Below. As in the United States, adoption of these politics of respectability by middle-class Caribbean leaders highlighted underlying class and gendered tensions among Black people, despite their shared goal to move toward nation-building and freedom from colonial rule. See Mosse, *Nationalism and Sexuality*; McClintock, *Imperial Leather*; Levine, *Prostitution, Race, and Politics* and *Gender and Empire*.

53. See Alexander, "Not Just (Any) Body." In an attempt to distance themselves from stereotypes of irresponsible working-class masculinity and promiscuous women's sexuality, many middle-class men and women availed themselves of opportunities of upward class and social mobility through education and training by the British on proper modes of respectable citizenship, moral rectitude, and the skills required to self-govern. For middle-class Afro-Caribbean men, patriotic and nationalist duty meant mastering respectable norms of the nuclear family and, once again, managing working-class Black women's sexuality. Many middle-class women, on the other hand, were trained in femininity, propriety, homemaking, etiquette, and the importance of fostering and guarding the nuclear family and children as the future of the nation.

54. As with their involvement in birth control campaigns, middle-class people's participation in the project of nationalism and its various tenets was largely complex, motivated in part by a strong desire to improve living conditions, increase development, and modernize, yet dramatically failing to challenge the "'naturalist' ideologies of racial order typified by the savage statelessness of Africans and by the civilized European governed by reason and rationality"; Hintzen, "Creoleness and Nationalism," 208.

55. Kamugisha, "Coloniality of Citizenship," 24–25. These radical political movements were largely transnational, influenced by pan-Africanist socialist ideologies, and worked alongside the Barbados Democratic Labour Party to oppose the political dominance of big business, liberalize employment policies, and democratize the economy. See Beckles, *History of Barbados*.

56. Unlike neighboring governments in the region, the Barbadian state, then led by Prime Minister Lloyd Sandiford of the Democratic Labour Party, refused to accept International Monetary Fund and World Bank structural adjustment policies in the early 1990s, which threatened to devalue Barbadian currency as a means to stabilize the economy. Instead, the government instituted a range of domestic protocols under the Social Partnership model to resolve the financial crises it faced at this time. Under these protocols, civic trust was built through the message that a common cultural heritage, social justice, and social stability were required for economic growth. As such, all public sector workers received a 10 percent pay cut, signaling a commitment to nationhood.

57. Derrida, *Dissemination*, 127. Building on Derrida's term, sociologists and science and technology studies scholars have mobilized the word to explore the possibilities and constraints of biotechnologies, pharmaceutical drugs, and digital frameworks and movements such as #MeToo, which generate productive spaces for feminist activism that are nonetheless enfolded in white neoliberal feminist agendas that foreclose intersectional feminism's radical ethos. See Persson, "Incorporating Pharmakon"; Pollock, *Medicating Race*; Wiens and MacDonald, "Feminist Futures."

58. Persson, "Incorporating Pharmakon," 49.

59. Pollock, *Medicating Race*, 170.

60. See Connell and Hunt, "HPV Vaccination Campaign"; Charles, "Mobilizing the Self-Governance"; Mamo, Nelson, and Clarke, "Producing and Protecting Risky Girlhoods"; Polzer and Knabe, "From Desire to Disease."

61. Connell and Hunt, "HPV Vaccination Campaign," 67. Despite the vaccine being offered to preteen boys and girls under Barbados's national vaccination program since 2015, popular and professional "medicomoralization" discourse around the vaccine and its promotion attaches disproportionately to women's sexuality; Connell and Hunt, "HPV Vaccination Campaign," 67.

62. De Barros, *Reproducing the British Caribbean*.

CHAPTER THREE. (HYPER)SEXUALITY, RESPECTABILITY,
AND THE LANGUAGE OF SUSPICION

Portions of chapter 3 appeared in an earlier form in "HPV Vaccination and Affective Suspicions in Barbados," *Feminist Formations* 30, no. 1 (Spring 2018): 46–70.

1. Mosse, *Nationalism and Sexuality*, 1.

2. Mosse, *Nationalism and Sexuality*.

3. See Alexander, "Redrafting Morality"; Olwig, "Struggle for Respectability"; Rheddock, "Women, Labour and Struggle"; Sheller, *Citizenship from Below*.

4. See Beckles, *Natural Rebels*; Besson, "Reputation and Respectability Reconsidered"; Sheller, "Quasheba, Mother, Queen"; Barrow, *Caribbean Portraits*. Common-law unions and other informal relationships that developed for Afro-Caribbeans during slavery continued after emancipation not as disrespectable forms of conduct but as traditional, creole social norms. The existence of visiting relationships—heterosexual unions wherein partners share an intimate relationship (often including children) but do not permanently reside together—as formal categories in Caribbean censuses from the 1970s also indicates a prevalent occurrence of these non–nuclear family forms and the state's acknowledgment of these widespread kinds of cohabitation that existed beyond heterosexual marriage. See also Robinson, "Properties of Citizens."

5. Wilson, *Crab Antics*.

6. Wilson, *Crab Antics*. See also Besson, "Reputation and Respectability Reconsidered" and *Martha Brae's Two Histories*; Freeman, *Entrepreneurial Selves*; Olwig, "Struggle for Respectability"; Sheller, "Quasheba, Mother, Queen."

7. Freeman, "'Reputation' of Neoliberalism," 254.

8. Agard-Jones, "Intimacy's Politics." For more on criticisms toward these respectability politics, see Kempadoo, *Sexing the Caribbean*; Thomas, *Modern Blackness*.

9. F. Smith, "Introduction," 2.

10. See Kempadoo, *Sexing the Caribbean*; Nixon, *Resisting Paradise*; Sharpe and Pinto, "Sweetest Taboo"; Smith, *Sex and the Citizen*.

11. See Bascomb, *In Plenty*; Cooper, *Noises in the Blood* and *Sound Clash*; Ellis, "Out and Bad"; Murray, *Flaming Souls*; Nixon, "Blackness, Resistance and Consciousness." Caribbeanists have extensively documented the challenges and forms of resistance toward a politics of respectability after independence through Caribbean musical traditions of dancehall and cultural traditions of Carnival. Carla Freeman builds on this

legacy of research, arguing that we might view the contentious paradigm of reputation/ respectability not only as being resisted but as shifting and being reworked in the context of increasing economic precarity and entrepreneurism in Barbados. See Freeman, *Entrepreneurial Selves*.

12. Mamo and Epstein, "Pharmaceuticalization of Sexual Risk," 162.

13. Alexander, "Redrafting Morality" and *Pedagogies of Crossing*.

14. Barriteau, "Theorizing Gender Systems" and *Political Economy of Gender*; Barriteau and Cobley, *Stronger, Surer, Bolder*.

15. Barriteau, "Engendering Development," 182.

16. Barriteau, *Political Economy of Gender*, 30.

17. See Alexander, *Pedagogies of Crossing*; Barrow, *Caribbean Portraits*; Chevannes, *Learning to Be a Man*; Kempadoo, *Sexing the Caribbean*; Lazarus, "This Is a Christian Nation."

18. Barriteau, "Theorizing Gender Systems," 196.

19. Barriteau, "Theorizing Gender Systems," 192.

20. Lazarus, "This Is a Christian Nation."

21. Lazarus, "This Is a Christian Nation," 121.

22. Lazarus, "This Is a Christian Nation," 123.

23. Mamo and Epstein, "Pharmaceuticalization of Sexual Risk," 155.

24. Mamo and Epstein, "Pharmaceuticalization of Sexual Risk."

25. Mamo and Epstein, "Pharmaceuticalization of Sexual Risk," 156. See also Biehl, "Pharmaceutical Governance."

26. Padmore, *Pan-Africanism or Communism?* Pan-Africanism reflects a plethora of cultural and political views that are broadly aimed toward decolonization, antiracism, and oppression.

27. Chapter 2 explored these fraught convergences between risk, surveillance, and biopolitics in more detail. For more on the surveillance of Black women's reproduction and colonial strategies to civilize, cure, and save Black and colonized people through the logics of science, social science, and biomedicine across the British empire, see Comaroff, "Diseased Heart of Africa"; De Barros, *Reproducing the British Caribbean*; Levine, *Prostitution, Race, and Politics*; Paton, "Enslaved Women and Slavery."

28. Henry, "Legal Gap Analysis."

29. Barriteau, "Theorizing Gender Systems," 194–95.

30. Barriteau, "Theorizing Gender Systems," 192.

31. Collier and Ong, "Global Assemblages," 4. As anthropologists have argued, global assemblages are intricately linked to long-standing transnational frames and global histories. Global assemblages, like neoliberal globalization, are thus not new in and of themselves but instead increasingly enfold emerging and developing technologies which affect and transform circuits and trajectories of change, exchange, and citizenship. See also Trouillot, *Global Transformations*. For more on pharmaceuticalization, see Mamo and Epstein, "Pharmaceuticalization of Sexual Risk."

32. See Collier and Ong, "Global Assemblages"; Horst and Miller, *Cell Phone*; Murray, *Flaming Souls*; Padilla, *Love and Globalization*.

33. Griffiths-Watson, "UNESCO/IBE Barbados Country Report." The Education

Sector Enhancement Programme, commonly referred to in Barbados as EDUTECH, is a multimillion-dollar government program initiated in 1999 with the financial assistance of the Caribbean Development Bank and the Inter-American Development Bank. The program aims to forge and sustain connections among the country's education and socioeconomic sectors by introducing new learning technologies, reforming the curriculum, training educational professionals, and upgrading facilities across public and private schools.

34. RRM, "Case Dismissed." This case was dismissed in July 2015.

35. C. Walcott, "Awright Den!"

36. L. Smith, "Sex Video with High School Students."

37. Guyana Times, "St. Rose's Students Undergoing Counselling."

38. Murray, *Flaming Souls.*

39. I draw this point from Carla Freeman, who emphasizes the challenge anthropologists face to explore and explicate the "deceptively familiar, even mundane" affective, economic, and social features of neoliberal life under globalization in Barbados and throughout the Caribbean; Freeman, *Entrepreneurial Selves*, 10.

40. Alexander, "Not Just (Any) Body," 6.

41. Brand, *Map to the Door of No Return*, 29.

42. Brand, *Map to the Door of No Return.*

43. See Alexander, "Not Just (Any) Body" and *Pedagogies of Crossing*; Kamugisha, "Coloniality of Citizenship"; King, *Island Bodies.*

44. Mamo and Epstein, "Pharmaceuticalization of Sexual Risk."

CHAPTER FOUR. CARE, EMBODIMENT, AND SENSED PROTECTION

1. *Oxford English Dictionary*, "sense."

2. Lorde, *Sister Outsider*, 37.

3. For more on the legacies of suspicion in African American communities in the wake of the Tuskegee syphilis experiments, see Dula, "African American Suspicion," 354–55; Washington, *Medical Apartheid*. For a more detailed discussion on coercive biomedical intervention in Puerto Rico, see Schoen, *Choice and Coercion*; Briggs, *Reproducing Empire.*

4. Moraga and Anzaldúa, "Entering the Lives of Others," 19.

5. Lorde, *Uses of the Erotic*, 56

6. Engaging Lorde, queer Afro-Caribbean diasporic scholars generatively suggest we might extend these popularly cited claims about the principle of eros and the erotic beyond the category of woman to interrogate more closely the lived anticolonial, anti-imperialist imperatives and experiences of racialized peoples (and possibilities of peoples) of the African diaspora by attending to the productive tensions that exist across the socioeconomic, political, cultural, spiritual, and sensual parts and desires in the feminine in each of us. See Gill, *Erotic Islands*; Tinsley, *Thiefing Sugar.*

7. Carabotti et al., "Gut-Brain Axis."

8. Wilson, *Gut Feminism*, 22.

9. Price, "Bodymind Problem."

10. Schalk, *Bodyminds Reimagined*, 6.

11. Judd, *Patient*.

12. Judd, *Patient*, 10.

13. Hartman, "Belly of the World," 168.

14. Ahmed and Stacey, *Thinking through the Skin*, 1.

15. Gilroy, *Against Race*, 46.

16. See Browne, *Dark Matters*; Hartman, *Scenes of Subjection* and "Belly of the World"; Patterson, *Slavery and Social Death*; Spillers, "Mama's Baby, Papa's Maybe."

17. Spillers, "Mama's Baby, Papa's Maybe," 67.

18. Spillers, "Mama's Baby, Papa's Maybe," 67.

19. Spillers, "Mama's Baby, Papa's Maybe," 67.

20. Chapter 3 contains further excerpts from Simone's interview, which highlight the multiple factors that underlie her suspicion toward the vaccine. In addition to her previous experiences with HPV, Simone describes how the vaccine symbolized a violent rather than protective force which, reminiscent of histories of control of Black women's bodies, could threaten her daughter's right to bodily autonomy and control as a sexual subject by instead turning the power for her body over to a pharmaceutical company.

21. Lorde, *Uses of the Erotic*, 37.

22. Murphy, "Unsettling Care."

23. I borrow this term from Hortense Spillers, who refers to an "American grammar" as the discursive parameters around which understandings of gender and race are constructed and made legible; Spillers, "Mama's Baby, Papa's Maybe," 68.

24. Hobart and Kneese, "Radical Care."

25. Nash, "Writing Black Beauty," 105.

CHAPTER FIVE. SUSPICION AND CERTAINTY

1. Parents I interviewed referred to Facebook groups such as UK Association of HPV Vaccine Injured Daughters and websites like Consider before Consent (www.cbc.help) and Gardasil Awareness NZ (www.ga-nz.com), none of which was still active as of 2019.

2. Gardasil Awareness NZ was created by a group of mothers who claim their daughters were injured by the vaccine.

3. Merck lists reported side effects of the quadrivalent vaccine as follows: "As with other vaccines, side effects that have been reported during general use include: swollen glands (neck, armpit, or groin), Guillain-Barré syndrome, headache, joint pain, aching muscles, unusual tiredness, weakness, or confusion, chills, bad stomach ache, muscle weakness, shortness of breath, generally feeling unwell, bleeding or bruising more easily than normal, and skin infection"; Merck & Co., "Gardasil Product Monograph," 61. Merck also states the following caveat: "This is not a complete list of side effects. For any unexpected effects while taking GARDASIL, contact your physician or pharmacist"; Merck & Co., "Gardasil Product Monograph," 61.

4. The term *post-truth* "relat[es] to or denot[es] circumstances in which objective facts are less influential in shaping political debate or public opinion than appeals to emotion and personal belief"; *Oxford English Dictionary*, "post-truth."

5. Hochschild, "Emotion Work."

6. Goldschmidt, "US Measles Cases."

7. The term *vaccine hesitancy* began to appear prominently in medical literature from 2011, largely replacing the use of *acceptance* and *compliance*. For scientific studies on the phenomenon, see Dubé et al., "Vaccine Hesitancy"; Salmon et al., "Vaccine Hesitancy"; Greenberg, Dubé, and Driedger, "Vaccine Hesitancy." For a sample of social science research on hesitancy, see Poltorak et al., "'MMR Talk' and Vaccination Choices"; Leach and Fairhead, *Vaccine Anxieties*; Goldenberg, "Public Misunderstanding of Science?"; Lawrence, Hausman, and Dannenberg, "Reframing Medicine's Publics."

8. Wakefield's fraudulent study was by no means the beginning of antivaccination sentiment. Much scholarship has analyzed the history of vaccination resistance in historical perspective across the United States and Europe. See Conis, *Vaccine Nation*; Durbach, *Bodily Matters*; Colgrove, *State of Immunity*. For more on Wakefield's role in fueling antivaccination propaganda, see Fitzpatrick, *MMR and Autism*; Largent, *Vaccine*.

9. Goldenberg, "Public Misunderstanding of Science?," 553.

10. See Offit, *Deadly Choices* and "Junk Science."

11. Leung, "Measles Cases Are Increasing."

12. Connolly et al., "Fake News."

13. Allcott and Gentzkow, "Social Media and Fake News," 213.

14. One such example is the meme with which I opened this book, which depicts a young Ugandan boy wearing a wry expression with text superimposed onto the image that reads, "So you mean to tell me some people turn down vaccinations?" Posted on the door of an immunization room in a polyclinic, this example highlights the affective resonance of viral productions and media in public health for both laypersons and medical professionals and the use value of this medium in health care campaigns.

15. *Oxford English Dictionary*, "certainty."

16. A plethora of opinion pieces on antivaccine websites like NaturalNews.com and the Anti-News Network suggest that Harper's claims are indicative of Merck conspiracies. See, for instance, Debbie, "Lead Developer of HPV Vaccine."

17. Harper and DeMars, "HPV Vaccines."

18. Hochschild, "Emotion Work," 551.

19. Hochschild, "Feeling around the World."

20. WAND, "Demystifying and Fighting Cervical Cancer."

21. WAND, "Demystifying and Fighting Cervical Cancer," 34.

22. WAND, "Demystifying and Fighting Cervical Cancer," 49.

23. WAND, "Demystifying and Fighting Cervical Cancer," 49.

24. Barriteau and Cobley, *Stronger, Surer, Bolder*.

25. See Hall, "Negotiating Caribbean Identities"; Benítez Rojo, *Repeating Island*.

26. Nelson, *Body and Soul*, 186.

27. Nelson, *Body and Soul*, 80.

28. Alexander, *Pedagogies of Crossing*, 190.

29. Hartman, *Lose Your Mother*, 6.

30. Hartman, *Lose Your Mother*, 6.

1. Hobart and Kneese, "Radical Care."

2. Loop News Barbados, "Rihanna-Funded Ventilators Coming Soon."

3. In April 2020, President Donald Trump also attempted to block the export of surgical masks manufactured by 3M by enacting the Defense Production Act. According to German Minister of the Interior Andreas Geisel, such seizes and export bans must be understood as "act[s] of modern piracy." Lough and Rinke, "'Act of Modern Piracy.'"

4. Ross and Jabkhiro, "French Doctor Apologizes."

5. Ross and Jabkhiro, "French Doctor Apologizes."

6. Inserm, "#FakeNews."

7. Alexander and Mohanty, "Cartographies of Knowledge."

8. Agard-Jones, "Bodies in the System," 185.

9. Médecins Sans Frontières (MSF) International, "DRC Ebola Outbreak."

Bibliography

Abbott, T. "PBS News: Government Funds Gardasil." Australian Government Department of Health, 2006. https://www.pbs.gov.au/info/news/2006/11/aust-govt-funds -gardasil.

Abu-Lughod, Lila. "The Romance of Resistance: Tracing Transformations of Power through Bedouin Women." *American Ethnologist* 17, no. 1 (1990): 41–55. https:// doi.org/10.1525/ae.1990.17.1.02a00030.

Agard-Jones, Vanessa. "Bodies in the System." *Small Axe* 17, no. 3 (2013): 182–92.

Agard-Jones, Vanessa. "Intimacy's Politics: New Directions in Caribbean Sexuality Studies." *Nieuwe West—Indische Gids* 85, nos. 3–4 (2011): 247.

Ahmed, Sara. "Affective Economies." *Social Text* 22, no. 2 (2004): 117–39.

Ahmed, Sara. *The Promise of Happiness*. Durham, NC: Duke University Press, 2010.

Ahmed, Sara, and Jackie Stacey. *Thinking through the Skin*. New York: Routledge, 2001.

Alexander, M. Jacqui. "Not Just (Any) Body Can Be a Citizen: The Politics of Law, Sexuality and Postcoloniality in Trinidad and Tobago and the Bahamas." *Feminist Review*, no. 48 (1994): 5. https://doi.org/10.2307/1395166.

Alexander, M. Jacqui. *Pedagogies of Crossing: Meditations on Feminism, Sexual Politics, Memory, and the Sacred*. Durham, NC: Duke University Press, 2005.

Alexander, M. Jacqui. "Redrafting Morality: The Postcolonial State and the Sexual Offences Bill of Trinidad and Tobago." In *Third World Women and the Politics of Feminism*, edited by Chandra Talpade Mohanty, Ann Russo, and Lourdes Torres, 133–52. Bloomington: Indiana University Press, 1991.

Alexander, M. Jacqui, and Chandra Talpade Mohanty. "Cartographies of Knowledge and Power: Transnational Feminism as Radical Praxis." In *Critical Transnational Feminist Praxis*, edited by Amanda Lock Swarr and Richa Nagar, 23–45. Albany: SUNY Press, 2010.

Allcott, Hunt, and Matthew Gentzkow. "Social Media and Fake News in the 2016 Election." *Journal of Economic Perspectives* 31, no. 2 (2017): 211–36. https://doi.org/10.1257 /jep.31.2.211.

Altink, Henrice. "'Fight TB with BCG': Mass Vaccination Campaigns in the British Caribbean, 1951–6." *Medical History* 58, no. 4 (2014): 475–97. https://doi.org/10.1017/mdh.2014.49.

Antrobus, Peggy. "Entrepreneurial Selves: Neoliberal Respectability and the Making of a Caribbean Middle Class." *Gender & Development* 23, no. 3 (2015): 559–62. https://doi.org/10.1080/13552074.2015.1112547.

Arthur, Owen. "Address by the Rt. Hon. Owen Arthur, Prime Minister of Barbados, at Caribbean Connect: A High-Level Symposium on the Single Market and Economy." Bridgetown, Barbados, Caribbean Community (CARICOM), 28 June 2006. https://caricom.org/address-by-the-rt-hon-owen-arthur-prime-minister-of-barbados-at-caribbean-connect-a-high-level-symposium-on-the-single-market-and-economy-28-30-june-2006-bridgetown-barbados/.

Barriteau, Eudine. *The Political Economy of Gender in the Twentieth-Century Caribbean.* Basingstoke, UK: Palgrave, 2001.

Barriteau, Eudine. "Theorizing Gender Systems and the Project of Modernity in the Twentieth-Century Caribbean." *Feminist Review*, no. 59 (Summer 1998): 186–210.

Barriteau, Eudine, and Alan Gregor Cobley. *Stronger, Surer, Bolder: Ruth Nita Barrow: Social Change and International Development.* Kingston: University Press of the West Indies, 2001.

Barriteau, V. Eudine. "Engendering Development or Gender Main-Streaming? A Critical Assessment from the Commonwealth Caribbean." In *Feminist Economics and the World Bank: History, Theory and Policy*, edited by Edith Kuiper and Drucilla K. Barker, 176–98. London: Routledge, 2006.

Barrow, Christine, ed. *Caribbean Portraits: Essays on Gender Ideologies and Identities.* Kingston: Ian Randle, 1998.

Barrow, Nita. "Women in the Front Line of Health Care." *Convergence* 15, no. 2 (1982): 82–84.

Bascomb, Lia T. *In Plenty and in Time of Need: Popular Culture and the Remapping of Barbadian Identity.* New Brunswick, NJ: Rutgers University Press, 2020.

Beck, Ulrich. *Risk Society: Towards a New Modernity.* London: Sage, 1992.

Beck, Ulrich. "The Terrorist Threat: World Risk Society Revisited." *Theory, Culture & Society* 19, no. 4 (2002): 39–55. https://doi.org/10.1177/0263276402019004003.

Beckles, Hilary. "Capitalism, Slavery and Caribbean Modernity." *Callaloo* 20, no. 4 (1997): 777–89. https://doi.org/10.1353/cal.1997.0070.

Beckles, Hilary. *A History of Barbados: From Amerindian Settlement to Nation-State.* New York: Cambridge University Press, 2007.

Beckles, Hilary. *Natural Rebels: A Social History of Enslaved Black Women in Barbados.* New Brunswick, NJ: Rutgers University Press, 1989.

Benítez Rojo, Antonio. *The Repeating Island: The Caribbean and the Postmodern Perspective*, 2nd ed. Durham, NC: Duke University Press, 1996.

Benjamin, Ruha. "Informed Refusal: Toward a Justice-Based Bioethics." *Science, Technology, & Human Values* 41, no. 6 (2016): 967.

Benjamin, Ruha. *People's Science: Bodies and Rights on the Stem Cell Frontier.* Stanford, CA: Stanford University Press, 2013.

Besson, Jean. *Martha Brae's Two Histories: European Expansion and Caribbean Culture-Building in Jamaica*. Chapel Hill: University of North Carolina Press, 2002.

Besson, Jean. "Reputation and Respectability Reconsidered: A New Perspective on Afro-Caribbean Peasant Women." In *Women and Change in the Caribbean: A Pan-Caribbean Perspective*, edited by Janet Henshall Momsen, 15–37. Bloomington: Indiana University Press, 1993.

Biehl, João. "Pharmaceutical Governance." In *Global Pharmaceuticals: Ethics, Markets, Practices*, edited by Adriana Petryna, Andrew Lakoff, and Andrew Kleinman, 206–39. Durham, NC: Duke University Press, 2006.

Biehl, João Guilherme. "Pharmaceuticalization: AIDS Treatment and Global Health Politics." *Anthropological Quarterly* 80, no. 4 (2007): 1083–126. https://doi.org/10.1353/anq.2007.0056.

Blake, Judith. *Family Structure in Jamaica: The Social Context of Reproduction*. New York: Free Press of Glencoe, 1961.

Bolland, O. Nigel. *The Politics of Labour in the British Caribbean: The Social Origins of Authoritarianism and Democracy in the Labour Movement*. Princeton, NJ: Markus Wiener, 2001.

Bonah, Christian. "'As Safe as Milk or Sugar Water': Perceptions of the Risks and Benefits of the BCG Vaccine in the 1920s and 1930s in France and Germany." In *The Risks of Medical Innovation: Risk Perception and Assessment in Historical Context*, edited by Thomas Schlich and Ulrich Tröhler, 66–86. New York: Routledge, 2006.

Bourbonnais, Nicole. "Class, Colour and Contraception: The Politics of Birth Control in Jamaica, 1938–1967." *Social and Economic Studies* 61, no. 3 (2012): 7–37.

Bourbonnais, Nicole. "Out of the Boudoir and into the Banana Walk: Birth Control and Reproductive Politics in the West Indies, 1930–1970." PhD diss., University of Pittsburgh, 2013. http://d-scholarship.pitt.edu/id/eprint/18314.

Brand, Dionne. *A Map to the Door of No Return: Notes to Belonging*. Toronto: Doubleday Canada, 2001.

Brandford, Albert. "PM's Case for Fingerprinting." *Nation News*, 17 March 2016. http://www.nationnews.com/nationnews/news/79054/pm-fingerprinting.

Brathwaite, George Christopher. "CARICOM and the Politics of Migration: Securitisation and the Free Movement of Community Nationals in Barbados." PhD diss., Newcastle University, 2014. http://hdl.handle.net/10443/2561.

Brennan, Teresa. *The Transmission of Affect*. Ithaca, NY: Cornell University Press, 2004.

Brereton, Bridget. "'All Ah We Is Not One': Historical and Ethnic Narratives in Pluralist Trinidad." *Global South* 4, no. 2 (2010): 218–38. https://doi.org/10.2979/globalsouth.4.2.218.

Briggs, Laura. *Reproducing Empire: Race, Sex, Science, and U.S. Imperialism in Puerto Rico*. Berkeley: University of California Press, 2002.

Brown, Nik. *Immunitary Life: A Biopolitics of Immunity*. London: Palgrave Macmillan, 2018.

Browne, David V. C. *Race, Class, Politics and the Struggle for Empowerment in Barbados, 1914–1937*. Miami: Ian Randle, 2012.

Browne, Simone. *Dark Matters: On the Surveillance of Blackness*. Durham, NC: Duke University Press, 2015.

Campt, Tina Marie. "Black Visuality and the Practice of Refusal." *Women and Performance: A Journal of Feminist Theory* 29, no. 1 (2019): 79–87. https://doi.org/10.1080
/0740770X.2019.1573625.

Carabotti, Marilia, Annunziata Scirocco, Maria Antonietta Maselli, and Carola Severi.
"The Gut-Brain Axis: Interactions between Enteric Microbiota, Central and Enteric
Nervous Systems." *Annals of Gastroenterology* 28, no. 2 (2015): 203–9.

Caribbean Community (CARICOM) Secretariat. "Revised Treaty of Chaguaramas Establishing the Caribbean Community Including the CARICOM Single Market and Economy." 2001. https://caricom.org/documents/4906-revised_treaty-text.pdf.

Caribbean Court of Justice. "Caribbean Court of Justice Application no. OA 002 of 2012
between Shanique Myrie and the State of Barbados and the State of Jamaica." 2013.
https://ccj.org/wp-content/uploads/2013/10/2013-CCJ-3-OJ.pdf.

Casper, Monica J., and Laura M. Carpenter. "Sex, Drugs, and Politics: The HPV Vaccine for
Cervical Cancer." *Sociology of Health and Illness* 30, no. 6 (2008): 886–99. https://
doi.org/10.1111/j.1467-9566.2008.01100.x.

CBC News. "P.E.I. Boys Offered HPV Vaccine." 19 April 2013. http://www.cbc.ca/news
/canada/prince-edward-island/p-e-i-boys-offered-hpv-vaccine-1.1339059.

Centers for Disease Control and Prevention (CDC). "HPV Vaccine Prevents HPV and Cancers That It Causes." Accessed 22 August 2019. https://www.cdc.gov/hpv/parents
/about-hpv-sp.html.

Challenger, Denise. "A Benign Place of Healing? The Contagious Diseases Hospital and
Medical Discipline in Post-Slavery Barbados." In *Health and Medicine in the Circum-
Caribbean, 1800–1968*, edited by Juanita De Barros, Steven Paul Palmer, and David
Wright, 98–117. New York: Routledge, 2009.

Chamberlain, Mary. *Empire and Nation-Building in the Caribbean: Barbados, 1937–66.*
New York: Palgrave Macmillan, 2010.

Charles, Nicole. "Mobilizing the Self-Governance of Pre-Damaged Bodies: Neoliberal Biological Citizenship and HPV Vaccination Promotion in Canada." *Citizenship Studies*
17, nos. 6–7 (2013): 770–84. https://doi.org/10.1080/13621025.2013.834128.

Charles-Soverall, Wayne, and Jamal Khan. "Social Partnership: New Public Management
Practice in Barbados." *African Journal of Public Administration and Management* 15,
no. 1 (2004): 22–36.

Chevannes, Barry. *Learning to Be a Man: Culture, Socialization and Gender Identity in
Five Caribbean Communities.* Barbados: University of the West Indies Press, 2001.

Clarke, Adele E., Janet K. Shim, Laura Mamo, Jennifer Ruth Fosket, and Jennifer R. Fish-
man. "Biomedicalization/A Theoretical and Substantive Introduction." In *Biomedicalization: Technoscience, Health, and Illness in the U.S.*, edited by Adele E. Clarke,
1–44. Durham, NC: Duke University Press, 2010.

Closser, Svea, Anat Rosenthal, Kenneth Maes, Judith Justice, Kelly Cox, Patricia A. Omid-
ian, Ismaila Zango Mohammed, Aminu Mohammed Dukku, Adam D. Koon, and
Laetitia Nyirazinyoye. "The Global Context of Vaccine Refusal: Insights from a Sys-
tematic Comparative Ethnography of the Global Polio Eradication Initiative." *Medical
Anthropology Quarterly* 30, no. 3 (2016): 321–41. https://doi.org/10.1111/maq.12254.

Clough, Patricia T. "The Affective Turn Political Economy, Biomedia and Bodies." *Theory, Culture & Society* 25, no. 1 (2008): 1–22. https://doi.org/10.1177/0263276407085156.

Colgrove, James Keith. *State of Immunity: The Politics of Vaccination in Twentieth-Century America*. Berkeley: University of California Press, 2006.

Collier, Stephen J., and Aihwa Ong. "Global Assemblages, Anthropological Problems." In *Global Assemblages: Technology, Politics, and Ethics as Anthropological Problems*, edited by Aihwa Ong and Stephen J. Collier, 3–21. Malden, MA: Blackwell, 2005.

Comaroff, Jean. "The Diseased Heart of Africa: Medicine, Colonialism, and the Black Body." In *Knowledge, Power, and Practice: The Anthropology of Medicine and Everyday Life*, edited by Shirley Lindenbaum and Margaret M. Lock, 305–29. Berkeley: University of California Press, 1993.

Conis, Elena. *Vaccine Nation: America's Changing Relationship with Immunization*. Chicago: University of Chicago Press, 2015.

Connell, Erin, and Alan Hunt. "The HPV Vaccination Campaign: A Project of Moral Regulation in an Era of Biopolitics." *Canadian Journal of Sociology/Cahiers Canadiens de Sociologie* 35, no. 1 (2010): 63–82.

Connolly, Kate, Angelique Chrisafis, Poppy McPherson, Stephanie Kirchgaessner, Benjamin Haas, Dominic Phillips, Elle Hunt, and Michael Safi. "Fake News: An Insidious Trend That's Fast Becoming a Global Problem." *The Guardian*, 2 December 2016. https://www.theguardian.com/media/2016/dec/02/fake-news-facebook-us-election-around-the-world.

Cooper, Carolyn C. *Noises in the Blood: Orality, Gender and the "Vulgar" Body of Jamaican Popular Culture*. London: Macmillan Caribbean, 1993.

Cooper, Carolyn C. *Sound Clash: Jamaican Dancehall Culture at Large*. New York: Palgrave Macmillan, 2004.

Cordel, Nadège, Camille Ragin, Monique Trival, Benoît Tressières, and Eustase Janky. "High-Risk Human Papillomavirus Cervical Infections among Healthy Women in Guadeloupe." *International Journal of Infectious Diseases* 41 (2015): 13–16. https://doi.org/10.1016/j.ijid.2015.10.012.

Council on Foreign Relations. "Map: Vaccine-Preventable Outbreaks." Council on Foreign Relations, 2015. http://www.cfr.org/interactives/GH_Vaccine_Map/index.html.

Cross, Malcolm. *Urbanization and Urban Growth in the Caribbean: An Essay on Social Change in Dependent Societies*. Cambridge: Cambridge University Press, 1979.

Cvetkovich, Ann. *An Archive of Feelings: Trauma, Sexuality, and Lesbian Public Cultures*. Durham, NC: Duke University Press, 2003.

DaCosta, Michael. *Colonial Origins, Institutions and Economic Performance in the Caribbean: Guyana and Barbados*. Washington, DC: International Monetary Fund, 2007. http://www.imf.org/external/pubs/ft/wp/2007/wp0743.pdf.

Das, Veena, and Ranendra Das. "Pharmaceuticals in Urban Ecologies: The Register of the Local." In *Global Pharmaceuticals: Ethics, Markets, Practices*, edited by Adriana Petryna, Andrew Lakoff, and Arthur Kleinman. Durham, NC: Duke University Press, 2006.

David. "The Hegemony of Trinidad Continues." *Barbados Underground* (blog), 11 May 2012. https://barbadosunderground.net/2012/05/10/the-hegemony-of-trinidad -continues/.

De Barros, Juanita. *Reproducing the British Caribbean: Sex, Gender, and Population Politics after Slavery.* Chapel Hill: University of North Carolina Press, 2014.

Debbie, Samantha. "Lead Developer of HPV Vaccine Admits It's a Giant, Deadly Scam." *Natural News*, 29 September 2016. https://www.naturalnews.com/055471_HPV _vaccines_whistleblower_vaccine_injury.html.

Delle, James A. *The Colonial Caribbean: Landscapes of Power in Jamaica's Plantation System.* Cambridge: Cambridge University Press, 2014.

Derrida, Jacques. *Dissemination.* Translated by Barbara Johnson. Chicago: University of Chicago Press, 1981.

Dubé, Eve, Caroline Laberge, Maryse Guay, and Paul Bramadat. "Vaccine Hesitancy." *Human Vaccines and Immunotherapeutics* 9, no. 8 (2013): 1763–73. https://doi.org /10.4161/hv.24657.

Dula, Annette. "African American Suspicion of the Healthcare System Is Justified: What Do We Do about It?" *Cambridge Quarterly of Healthcare Ethics: CQ* 3, no. 3 (1994): 347–57.

Durbach, Nadja. *Bodily Matters: The Anti-Vaccination Movement in England, 1853–1907.* Durham, NC: Duke University Press, 2005.

Edmonds, Juliet, and Cherita Girvan. "Child Care and Family Services in Barbados." *Social and Economic Studies* 22, no. 2 (1973): 229.

Ellis, Nadia. "Out and Bad: Toward a Queer Performance Hermeneutic in Jamaican Dancehall." *Small Axe* 15, no. 2 (35) (2011): 7–23. https://doi.org/10.1215/07990537 -1334212.

Fitzpatrick, Michael. *MMR and Autism: What Parents Need to Know.* London: Routledge, 2004.

Foucault, Michel. *The History of Sexuality.* New York: Vintage Books, 1990.

Freeman, Carla. *Entrepreneurial Selves: Neoliberal Respectability and the Making of a Caribbean Middle Class.* Durham, NC: Duke University Press, 2014.

Freeman, Carla. "The 'Reputation' of Neoliberalism." *American Ethnologist* 34, no. 2 (2007): 252–67. https://doi.org/10.1525/ae.2007.34.2.252.

Garcia-Rojas, Claudia. "(Un)Disciplined Futures: Women of Color Feminism as a Disruptive to White Affect Studies." *Journal of Lesbian Studies* 21, no. 3 (2017): 254–71. https://doi.org/10.1080/10894160.2016.1159072.

Gavi Alliance. "Vaccine-Preventable Disease Outbreaks." *Vaccine-Preventable Disease Outbreaks Map* (blog), 2017. http://www.vaccineswork.org/vaccine-preventable -disease-outbreaks/.

Ghinai, Isaac, Chris Willott, Ibrahim Dadari, and Heidi J. Larson. "Listening to the Rumours: What the Northern Nigeria Polio Vaccine Boycott Can Tell Us Ten Years On." *Global Public Health* 8, no. 10 (2013): 1138–50. https://doi.org/10.1080/17441692 .2013.859720.

Gill, Lyndon K. *Erotic Islands: Art and Activism in the Queer Caribbean.* Durham, NC: Duke University Press, 2018.

Gilman, Sander L. "Black Bodies, White Bodies: Toward an Iconography of Female Sexuality in Late Nineteenth-Century Art, Medicine, and Literature." *Critical Inquiry* 12, no. 1 (1985): 204–42.

Gilroy, Paul. *Against Race: Imagining Political Culture beyond the Color Line.* Cambridge, MA: Belknap Press of Harvard University Press, 2000.

Girvan, Norman. "The 'Real' Immigration Problem in Barbados, CFHA." *Caribbean Political Economy* (blog), 17 June 2009. http://www.normangirvan.info/the-real-immigration-problem-in-barbados-cfha/.

Goldenberg, Maya J. "Public Misunderstanding of Science? Reframing the Problem of Vaccine Hesitancy." *Perspectives on Science* 24, no. 5 (2016): 552–81. https://doi.org/10.1162/POSC_a_00223.

Goldschmidt, Debra. "US Measles Cases Reach Highest Number in Nearly Three Decades, CDC Says." CNN, 30 May 2019. https://www.cnn.com/2019/05/30/health/us-measles-highest-since-1994-cdc-bn/index.html.

Gorton, K. "Theorizing Emotion and Affect: Feminist Engagements." *Feminist Theory* 8, no. 3 (2007): 333–48. https://doi.org/10.1177/1464700107082369.

Green, Cecilia A. "The 1938–1939 Moyne Commission in Barbados: Investigating the Status of Children." *Atlantic Studies* 11, no. 4 (2014): 515–35. https://doi.org/10.1080/14788810.2014.935639.

Greenberg, Joshua, Eve Dubé, and Michelle Driedger. "Vaccine Hesitancy: In Search of the Risk Communication Comfort Zone." *PLoS Currents Outbreaks*, 3 March 2017. https://doi.org/10.1371/currents.outbreaks.0561a011117a1d1f9596e24949e8690b.

Greene, Jeremy A. "Therapeutic Infidelities: 'Noncompliance' Enters the Medical Literature, 1955–1975." *Social History of Medicine* 17, no. 3 (2004): 327–43. https://doi.org/10.1093/shm/17.3.327.

Gregg, Melissa, and Gregory J. Seigworth, eds. *The Affect Theory Reader.* Durham, NC: Duke University Press, 2010.

Grewal, Inderpal, and Caren Kaplan. "Postcolonial Studies and Transnational Feminist Practices." *Jouvert: A Journal of Postcolonial Studies* 5, no. 1 (2000).

Grewal, Inderpal, and Caren Kaplan, eds. *Scattered Hegemonies: Postmodernity and Transnational Feminist Practices.* Minneapolis: University of Minnesota Press, 1994.

Griffiths-Watson, Wendy. "UNESCO/IBE Barbados Country Report—Curriculum Development." Sub-Regional Seminar on Curriculum Development for "Learning to Live Together," Havana, Cuba, UNESCO/IBE, May 2001. http://www.ibe.unesco.org/fileadmin/user_upload/archive/curriculum/Caribbean/CaribbeanPdf/barbados.pdf.

Grossberg, Lawrence. "History, Politics and Postmodernism: Stuart Hall and Cultural Studies." *Journal of Communication Inquiry* 10, no. 2 (1986): 61–77. https://doi.org/10.1177/019685998601000205.

Guyana Times. "St. Rose's Students Undergoing Counselling." 13 October 2014. http://www.guyanatimesgy.com/2014/10/13/st-roses-students-undergoing-counselling.

Hall, Stuart. "The Local and the Global: Globalization and Ethnicity." In *Culture, Globalization, and the World-System: Contemporary Conditions for the Representation of Identity*, edited by Anthony D. King, 19–39. Minneapolis: University of Minnesota Press, 1997.

Hall, Stuart. "Negotiating Caribbean Identities." In *New Caribbean Thought: A Reader*, edited by Brian Meeks and Folke Lindahl, 24–39. Kingston: University of West Indies Press, 2001.

Haraway, Donna. *Staying with the Trouble: Making Kin in the Chthulucene*. Durham, NC: Duke University Press, 2016.

Harper, Diane M., and Leslie R. DeMars. "HPV Vaccines—A Review of the First Decade." *Gynecologic Oncology* 146, no. 1 (2017): 196–204. https://doi.org/10.1016/j.ygyno.2017.04.004.

Hartman, Saidiya V. "The Belly of the World: A Note on Black Women's Labors." *Souls* 18, no. 1 (2016): 166–73. https://doi.org/10.1080/10999949.2016.1162596.

Hartman, Saidiya V. *Lose Your Mother: A Journey along the Atlantic Slave Route*. New York: Farrar, Straus and Giroux, 2007.

Hartman, Saidiya V. *Scenes of Subjection: Terror, Slavery, and Self-Making in Nineteenth-Century America*. New York: Oxford University Press, 1997.

Henry, Ruth. "A Legal Gap Analysis of Adolescent Sexual and Reproductive Health and Rights in Barbados." UNFPA, 2011. https://caribbean.unfpa.org/webdav/site/caribbean/shared/publications/2011/Barbados/SRH/Legal%20Gap%20Analysis%20ASRH%20Barbados.pdf.

Higginbotham, Evelyn Brooks. *Righteous Discontent: The Women's Movement in the Black Baptist Church, 1880–1920*. Cambridge, MA: Harvard University Press, 1993.

Hine, Darlene Clark. "Rape and the Inner Lives of Black Women in the Middle West." *Signs* 14, no. 4 (1989): 912–20.

Hintzen, Percy. "Creoleness and Nationalism in Guyanese Anticolonialism and Postcolonial Formation." *Small Axe* 8, no. 1 (2004): 107–22.

Hobart, Hiʻilei Julia Kawehipuaakahaopulani, and Tamara Kneese. "Radical Care Survival Strategies for Uncertain Times." *Social Text* 38, no. 1 (142) (2020): 1–16. https://doi.org/10.1215/01642472-7971067.

Hochschild, Arlie. "Feeling around the World." *Contexts* 7, no. 2 (2008): 80. https://doi.org/10.1525/ctx.2008.7.2.80.

Hochschild, Arlie Russell. "Emotion Work, Feeling Rules, and Social Structure." *American Journal of Sociology* 85, no. 3 (1979): 551–75.

Horst, Heather A., and Daniel. Miller, eds. *The Cell Phone: An Anthropology of Communication*. Oxford: Berg, 2006.

HPV Information Centre. "Human Papillomavirus and Related Diseases in Barbados." 17 June 2019. http://www.hpvcentre.net/statistics/reports/BRB.pdf.

Hutton, Maisha. "Mobilising Civil Society Improving Cancer Outcomes PAHO Women's Cancers Meeting." Healthy Caribbean Coalition, 11 May 2016. http://www.paho.org/hq/index.php?option=com_docman&task=doc_download&gid=34630&Itemid=270&lang=en.

Ifill, Mellissa. "The Transformation of the Sphere of Governance in Developing Societies: Examining Guyana's Transformation." Sir Arthur Lewis Conference, University of the West Indies Cave Hill Barbados, 2003.

Inserm. "#FakeNews." Twitter, 2 April 2020. https://twitter.com/inserm/status/1245686267188256768.

Jaggar, Alison M. "Love and Knowledge: Emotion in Feminist Epistemology." *Inquiry* 32, no. 2 (1989): 151–76. https://doi.org/10.1080/00201748908602185.

Jones, Cecily. "Human Weeds, Not Fit to Breed?: African Caribbean Women and Reproductive Disparities in Britain." *Critical Public Health* 23, no. 1 (2013): 49–61. https://doi.org/10.1080/09581596.2012.761676.

Judd, Bettina. *Patient: Poems*. New York: Black Lawrence Press, 2014.

Kamugisha, A. "The Coloniality of Citizenship in the Contemporary Anglophone Caribbean." *Race and Class* 49, no. 2 (2007): 20–40. https://doi.org/10.1177/0306396807082856.

Keller, Richard C. "Geographies of Power, Legacies of Mistrust: Colonial Medicine in the Global Present." *Historical Geography* 34 (2006): 26–48.

Kempadoo, Kamala. *Sexing the Caribbean: Gender, Race, and Sexual Labor*. New York: Routledge, 2004.

King, Rosamond S. *Island Bodies: Transgressive Sexualities in the Caribbean Imagination*. Gainesville: University Press of Florida, 2014.

King, Tiffany Lethabo. *The Black Shoals: Offshore Formations of Black and Native Studies*. Durham, NC: Duke University Press, 2019.

LaFont, Suzanne. "Very Straight Sex: The Development of Sexual Mores in Jamaica." *Journal of Colonialism and Colonial History* 2, no. 3 (2001). https://doi.org/10.1353/cch.2001.0051.

Largent, Mark A. *Vaccine: The Debate in Modern America*. Baltimore, MD: Johns Hopkins University Press, 2012.

Larson, Heidi J., Louis Z. Cooper, Juhani Eskola, Samuel L. Katz, and Scott Ratzan. "Addressing the Vaccine Confidence Gap." *Lancet* 378, no. 9790 (2011): 526–35. https://doi.org/10.1016/S0140-6736(11)60678-8.

Lawrence, Heidi, Bernice Hausman, and Clare Dannenberg. "Reframing Medicine's Publics: The Local as a Public of Vaccine Refusal." *Journal of Medical Humanities* 35, no. 2 (2014): 111–29. https://doi.org/10.1007/s10912-014-9278-4.

Lazarus, Latoya. "This Is a Christian Nation: Gender and Sexuality in Processes of Constitutional and Legal Reform in Jamaica." *Social and Economic Studies* 61, no. 3 (2012): 117–43.

Leach, Melissa, and James Fairhead. *Vaccine Anxieties: Global Science, Child Health, and Society*. Sterling, VA: Earthscan, 2007.

Leung, Hillary. "Measles Cases Are Increasing amid 'Complacency,' U.N. Warns." *Time*, 1 March 2019. https://time.com/5541677/measles-increase-globally-unicef/.

Levine, Philippa, ed. *Gender and Empire*. New York: Oxford University Press, 2004.

Levine, Philippa. *Prostitution, Race, and Politics: Policing Venereal Disease in the British Empire*. New York: Routledge, 2003.

Levy, Jonathan. *Freaks of Fortune: The Emerging World of Capitalism and Risk in America*. Cambridge, MA: Harvard University Press, 2012.

Lewis, Linden. "The Contestation of Race in Barbadian Society and the Camouflage of Conservatism." In *New Caribbean Thought: A Reader*, edited by Brian Meeks and Folke Lindahl, 144–95. Kingston: University of West Indies Press, 2001.

Lock, Margaret M., and Vinh-Kim Nguyen. "Biomedical Technologies in Practice." In *An*

Anthropology of Biomedicine, edited by Margaret Lock and Vinh-Kim Nguyen, 15–32. Malden, MA: Wiley-Blackwell, 2010.

Loop News Barbados. "Rihanna-Funded Ventilators Coming Soon, Others Seized by US." 5 April 2020. http://www.loopnewsbarbados.com/content/rihanna-donated-ventilators-coming-soon-others-seized-us.

Lorde, Audre. *Sister Outsider: Essays and Speeches*. Berkeley, CA: Crossing Press, 2007.

Lorde, Audre Geraldine. *Uses of the Erotic: The Erotic as Power*. Berkeley, CA: Ten Speed Press, 1984.

Lough, Richard, and Andreas Rinke. "'Act of Modern Piracy': U.S. Slammed amid Global Scramble over Face Masks." Reuters, 3 April 2020. https://globalnews.ca/news/6775423/coroanvirus-global-face-mask-competition/.

Magnello, Eileen. "The Introduction of Mathematical Statistics into Medical Research: The Roles of Karl Pearson, Major Greenwood, and Austin Bradford Hill." In *The Road to Medical Statistics*, edited by Eileen Magnello and Anne Hardy, 95–123. Amsterdam: Rodopi, 2002.

Mamo, Laura, and Steven Epstein. "The Pharmaceuticalization of Sexual Risk: Vaccine Development and the New Politics of Cancer Prevention." *Social Science and Medicine* 101 (2014): 155–65. https://doi.org/10.1016/j.socscimed.2013.11.028.

Mamo, Laura, Amber Nelson, and Aleia Clarke. "Producing and Protecting Risky Girlhoods." In *Three Shots at Prevention: The HPV Vaccine and the Politics of Medicine's Simple Solutions*, edited by Keith Wailoo, Julie Livingston, Steven Epstein, and Robert Aronowitz, 121–45. Baltimore, MD: Johns Hopkins University Press, 2010.

Marks, Lara. "Assessing the Risk and Safety of the Pill: Maternal Mortality and the Pill." In *The Risks of Medical Innovation: Risk Perception and Assessment in Historical Context*, edited by Thomas Schlich and Ulrich Tröhler, 170–85. London: Routledge, 2006.

Maskovsky, Jeff. "Do People Fail Drugs, or Do Drugs Fail People? The Discourse of Adherence." *Transforming Anthropology* 13, no. 2 (2005): 136–42. https://doi.org/10.1525/tran.2005.13.2.136.

Massiah, Joycelin. "The Population of Barbados: Demographic Development and Population Policy in a Small Island State." Thesis, University of the West Indies, 1981.

Massumi, Brian. *Parables for the Virtual: Movement, Affect, Sensation*. Durham, NC: Duke University Press, 2002.

McClintock, Anne. *Imperial Leather: Race, Gender, and Sexuality in the Colonial Contest*. New York: Routledge, 1995.

McGranahan, Carole. "Theorizing Refusal: An Introduction." *Cultural Anthropology* 31, no. 3 (2016): 319–25. https://doi.org/10.14506/ca31.3.01.

Médecins sans frontières (MSF) International. "DRC Ebola Outbreak Response Struggling One Year On." 19 May 2020. https://www.msf.org/drc-ebola-outbreak-response-struggling-one-year.

Merck & Co. "GARDASIL Product Monograph, Part III: Consumer Information." M2017. https://www.merck.ca/static/pdf/GARDASIL-CI_E.pdf.

Ministry of Labour and Immigration. "Comprehensive Review of Immigration Policy and

Proposals for Legislative Reform." October 2009. https://barbadosunderground.files
.wordpress.com/2009/10/green_paper_on_immigration_policy.pdf.

Moraga, Cherríe. "Catching Fire: Preface to the Fourth Edition." In *This Bridge Called
My Back: Writings by Radical Women of Color*, edited by Cherríe Moraga and Gloria
Anzaldúa, xv–xxv. Albany: SUNY Press, 2015.

Moraga, Cherríe, and Gloria Anzaldúa. "Entering the Lives of Others: Theory in the
Flesh." In *This Bridge Called My Back: Writings by Radical Women of Color*, edited
by Cherríe Moraga and Gloria Anzaldúa, 19. Albany, NY: SUNY Press, 2015.

Moraga, Cherríe, and Gloria Anzaldúa, eds. *This Bridge Called My Back: Writings by
Radical Women of Color*. Albany: SUNY Press, 2015.

Morgensen, Scott Lauria. *Spaces between Us: Queer Settler Colonialism and Indigenous
Decolonization*. Minneapolis: University of Minnesota Press, 2011.

Morris, Susana M. *Close Kin and Distant Relatives: The Paradox of Respectability in
Black Women's Literature*. Charlottesville: University of Virginia Press, 2014.

Mosse, George L. *Nationalism and Sexuality: Respectability and Abnormal Sexuality in
Modern Europe*. New York: Howard Fertig, 1985.

Murphy, Michelle. "Unsettling Care: Troubling Transnational Itineraries of Care in Feminist Health Practices." *Social Studies of Science* 45, no. 5 (2015): 717–37. https://doi
.org/10.1177/0306312715589136.

Murray, David. *Flaming Souls: Homosexuality, Homophobia, and Social Change in Barbados*. Toronto: University of Toronto Press, 2012.

Nash, Jennifer C. "Writing Black Beauty." *Signs: Journal of Women in Culture and Society*
45, no. 1 (2019): 101–22. https://doi.org/10.1086/703497.

Naus, M. "What Do We Know about How to Improve Vaccine Uptake?" *Canada Communicable Disease Report* 41, no. S3 (2015): 6.

Nelson, Alondra. *Body and Soul: The Black Panther Party and the Fight against Medical
Discrimination*. Minneapolis: University of Minnesota Press, 2011.

Newstead, Clare. "Regional Governmentality: Neoliberalization and the Caribbean Community Single Market and Economy." *Singapore Journal of Tropical Geography* 30,
no. 2 (2009): 158–73. https://doi.org/10.1111/j.1467-9493.2009.00364.x.

Nixon, Angelique V. "Blackness, Resistance and Consciousness in Dancehall Culture."
Black Renaissance/Renaissance Noire 9, nos. 2–3 (2009): 190–99.

Nixon, Angelique V. *Resisting Paradise: Tourism, Diaspora, and Sexuality in Caribbean
Culture*. Jackson: University Press of Mississippi, 2015.

Offit, Paul A. *Deadly Choices: How the Anti-Vaccine Movement Threatens Us All*. New
York: Basic Books/Perseus Books Group, 2011.

Offit, Paul A. "Junk Science Isn't a Victimless Crime." *Wall Street Journal*, 11 January 2011.
https://www.wsj.com/articles/SB10001424052748703779704576073744290909186.

Olwig, Karen Fog. "The Struggle for Respectability: Methodism and Afro-Caribbean Culture on 19th Century Nevis." *New West Indian Guide/Nieuwe West-Indische Gids* 64,
nos. 3–4 (1990): 93–114. https://doi.org/10.1163/13822373-90002018.

Oxford English Dictionary Online. "Certainty, n." Accessed 29 April 2019. http://www
.oed.com/view/Entry/29979.

Oxford English Dictionary Online. "Post-Truth, adj." Accessed 22 May 2019. http://www
.oed.com/view/Entry/58609044.

Oxford English Dictionary Online. "Sense, n." In *Oxford English Dictionary*. Accessed 18
April 2019. https://www.oed.com/view/Entry/17595.

Oxford English Dictionary Online. "Suspicion, n." Accessed 5 November 2020. https://
www.oed.com/view/Entry/195179.

Padilla, Mark. *Love and Globalization: Transformations of Intimacy in the Contemporary
World*. Nashville, TN: Vanderbilt University Press, 2007.

Padmore, George. *Pan-Africanism or Communism? The Coming Struggle for Africa*. London: Dennis Dobson, 1971.

Parker, Jason C. *Brother's Keeper: The United States, Race, and Empire in the British Caribbean, 1937–1962*. New York: Oxford University Press, 2008.

Paton, Diana. "Enslaved Women and Slavery before and after 1807." *History in Focus* 12
(2007). https://archives.history.ac.uk/history-in-focus/Slavery/articles/paton.html.

Patterson, Orlando. *Slavery and Social Death: A Comparative Study*. Cambridge, MA:
Harvard University Press, 1982.

Paugh, Katherine. "The Politics of Childbearing in the British Caribbean and the Atlantic
World during the Age of Abolition, 1776–1838." *Past and Present* 221, no. 1 (2013):
119–60. https://doi.org/10.1093/pastj/gtt011.

Paugh, Katherine. *The Politics of Reproduction: Race, Medicine, and Fertility in the Age of
Abolition*. New York: Oxford University Press, 2017.

Persson, Asha. "Incorporating Pharmakon: HIV, Medicine, and Body Shape Change." *Body
and Society* 10, no. 4 (2004): 45–67. https://doi.org/10.1177/1357034X04047855.

Petryna, Adriana. *Life Exposed: Biological Citizens after Chernobyl*. Princeton, NJ: Princeton University Press, 2002.

Philip, Kavita. "Keep on Copyin' in the Free World? Genealogies of the Postcolonial Pirate
Figure." In *Postcolonial Piracy: Media Distribution and Cultural Production in the
Global South*, edited by Anja Schwarz and Lars Eckstein, 149–78. New York: Blooms-
bury Academic, 2014.

Philip, Marlene NourbeSe. *Caribana: African Roots and Continuities: Race, Space and
the Poetics of Moving*. Toronto: Poui Publications, 1996.

Pollock, Anne. *Medicating Race: Heart Disease and Durable Preoccupations with Difference*. Durham, NC: Duke University Press, 2012.

Poltorak, Mike, Melissa Leach, Jackie Cassell, and James Fairhead. "'MMR Talk' and Vaccination Choices: An Ethnographic Study in Brighton." *Social Science and Medicine* 61,
no. 3 (2005): 709–19.

Polzer, Jessica C., and Susan M. Knabe. "From Desire to Disease: Human Papillomavirus
(HPV) and the Medicalization of Nascent Female Sexuality." *Journal of Sex Research*
49, no. 4 (2012): 344–52. https://doi.org/10.1080/00224499.2011.644598.

Price, Margaret. "The Bodymind Problem and the Possibilities of Pain." *Hypatia* 30, no. 1
(2015): 268–84.

Puri, Shalini. *The Caribbean Postcolonial: Social Equality, Post-Nationalism, and Cultural Hybridity*. New York: Palgrave Macmillan, 2004.

Putnam, Lara. "Global Child-Saving, Transatlantic Maternalism, and the Pathologization of Caribbean Childhood, 1920s–1940s." *Atlantic Studies/Global Currents* 11, no. 4 (2014): 491–514.

Rapp, Rayna. *Testing Women, Testing the Fetus: The Social Impact of Amniocentesis in America*. London: Routledge, 1999.

Reddit. "Make This Skeptical Kid into a Meme, STAT! (Took This Photo during My Medical Trip to Uganda This Month)." 20 June 2012. https://www.reddit.com/r/pics/comments/vc0c9/make_this_skeptical_kid_into_a_meme_stat_took/.

Redfield, Peter. "Doctors, Borders, and Life in Crisis." *Cultural Anthropology* 20, no. 3 (2005): 328–61. https://doi.org/10.1525/can.2005.20.3.328.

Republic Bank Limited. "Subsidiaries." Republic Bank, 2018. https://republicbarbados.com/about/subsidiaries.

Rheddock, Rhoda. "Women, Labour and Struggle in 20th Century Trinidad and Tobago: 1980–1984." PhD diss., University of Amsterdam, 1984.

Roberts, Dorothy. "The Social Immorality of Health in the Gene Age: Race, Disability, and Inequality." In *Against Health: How Health Became the New Morality*, edited by Jonathan Metzl and Anna Rutherford Kirkland, 61–71. New York: New York University Press, 2010.

Robinson, Tracy. "The Properties of Citizens." *Du Bois Review: Social Science Research on Race* 10, no. 2 (2013): 425–46. https://doi.org/10.1017/S1742058X13000209.

Rose, Nikolas S. *The Politics of Life Itself: Biomedicine, Power, and Subjectivity in the Twenty-First Century*. Princeton, NJ: Princeton University Press, 2007.

Rose, Nikolas S., and Carl Novas. "Biological Citizenship." In *Global Assemblages: Technology, Politics, and Ethics as Anthropological Problems*, edited by Aihwa Wong and Stephen J. Collier, 439–63. Malden, MA: Blackwell, 2005.

Ross, Aaron, and Juliette Jabkhiro. "French Doctor Apologises for Suggesting COVID-19 Treatment Be Tested in Africa," Reuters, 3 April 2020. https://www.reuters.com/article/us-health-coronavirus-africa-apology/french-doctor-apologises-for-suggesting-covid-19-treatment-be-tested-in-africa-idUSKBN21L2MS.

Rowley, Michelle V. *Feminist Advocacy and Gender Equity in the Anglophone Caribbean: Envisioning a Politics of Coalition*. London: Routledge, 2013.

RRM. "Case Dismissed." *Nation News*, 3 July 2015. http://www.nationnews.com/nationnews/news/69439/dismissed.

Rusnock, Andrea. "'The Merchant's Logick': Numerical Debates over Smallpox Inoculation in Eighteenth-Century England." In *The Road to Medical Statistics*, edited by Eileen Magnello and Anne Hardy, 37–54. Amsterdam: Rodopi, 2002.

Sagicor Life. "Sagicor and the Barbados Cancer Society Launches a Rebranded Globeathon as Gynathon to End Women's Gynaecological Cancers." Sagicor Life press release, 12 June 2019.

Saldanha, Arun. "The Political Geography of Many Bodies." In *The SAGE Handbook of Political Geography*, edited by Kevin Cox, Murray Low, and Jenny Robinson, 323–34. London: Sage, 2008.

Salmon, Daniel A., Matthew Z. Dudley, Jason M. Glanz, and Saad B. Omer. "Vaccine Hesitancy: Causes, Consequences, and a Call to Action." *Vaccine* 33 (2015): D66–D71.

Saunders, Alphea. "HPV Vaccine Administered to 309 Girls in 4 Schools—Tufton." *Ja-*

maica Observer, 4 October 2017. http://www.jamaicaobserver.com/article
/20171004/ARTICLE/171009842.

Schalk, Samantha Dawn. *Bodyminds Reimagined: (Dis)Ability, Race, and Gender in Black Women's Speculative Fiction*. Durham, NC: Duke University Press, 2018.

Schlich, Thomas. "Risk and Medical Innovation: A Historical Perspective." In *The Risks of Medical Innovation: Risk Perception and Assessment in Historical Context*, edited by Thomas Schlich and Ulrich Tröhler, 1–17. London: Routledge, 2006.

Schoen, Johanna. *Choice and Coercion: Birth Control, Sterilization, and Abortion in Public Health and Welfare*. Chapel Hill: University of North Carolina Press, 2005.

Sedgwick, Eve Kosofsky, and Adam Frank. *Touching Feeling: Affect, Pedagogy, Performativity*. Durham, NC: Duke University Press, 2003.

Segal, Aaron. *Population Policies in the Caribbean*. Lexington, MA: Lexington Books, 1975.

Seymour, Susan. "Resistance." *Anthropological Theory* 6, no. 3 (2006): 303–21. https://doi.org/10.1177/1463499606066890.

Sharpe, Christina Elizabeth. *In the Wake: On Blackness and Being*. Durham, NC: Duke University Press, 2016.

Sharpe, Jenny, and Samantha Pinto. "The Sweetest Taboo: Studies of Caribbean Sexualities; A Review Essay." *Signs* 32, no. 1 (2006): 247–74. https://doi.org/10.1086/505541.

Sheller, Mimi. *Citizenship from Below: Erotic Agency and Caribbean Freedom*. Durham, NC: Duke University Press, 2012.

Sheller, Mimi. "Quasheba, Mother, Queen: Black Women's Public Leadership and Political Protest in Post-Emancipation Jamaica, 1834–65." *Slavery and Abolition* 19, no. 3 (1998): 90–117. https://doi.org/10.1080/01440399808575257.

Shohat, Ella. "Notes on the 'Post-Colonial.'" *Social Text*, nos. 31–32 (1992): 99–113. https://doi.org/10.2307/466220.

Shohat, Ella. *Talking Visions: Multicultural Feminism in Transnational Age*. Cambridge, MA: MIT Press, 1998.

Simpson, Audra. *Mohawk Interruptus: Political Life across the Borders of Settler States*. Durham, NC: Duke University Press, 2014.

Slavin, Stephen L., and Richard E. Bilsborrow. "The Barbados Family Planning Association and Fertility Decline in Barbados." *Studies in Family Planning* 5, no. 10 (1974): 325–32.

Smith, Faith. "Introduction: Sexing the Citizen." In *Sex and the Citizen: Interrogating the Caribbean*, edited by Faith Smith, 1–17. Charlottesville: University of Virginia Press, 2011.

Smith, Leroy. "Sex Video with High School Students Goes Viral; Education Min. Disturbed." *Inewsguyana*, 6 October 2014. http://www.inewsguyana.com/sex-video-with-high-school-students-goes-viral-education-min-disturbed/.

Snelgrove, Corey, Rita Dhamoon, and Jeff Corntassel. "Unsettling Settler Colonialism: The Discourse and Politics of Settlers, and Solidarity with Indigenous Nations." *Decolonization: Indigeneity, Education & Society* 3, no. 2 (2014). https://jps.library.utoronto.ca/index.php/des/article/view/21166.

Sobo, Elisa J. "Theorizing (Vaccine) Refusal: Through the Looking Glass." *Cultural Anthropology* 31, no. 3 (2016): 342–50. https://doi.org/10.14506/ca31.3.04.

Spillers, Hortense. "Mama's Baby, Papa's Maybe: An American Grammar Book." *Diacritics* 17 (1987): 65–81.

Stycos, J. Mayone, and Jurt W. Back. *The Control of Human Fertility in Jamaica*. Ithaca, NY: Cornell University Press, 1964.

Sunder Rajan, Kaushik. *Biocapital: The Constitution of Postgenomic Life*. Durham, NC: Duke University Press, 2006.

Sunder Rajan, Kaushik. "Subjects of Speculation: Emergent Life Sciences and Market Logics in the United States and India." *American Anthropologist* 107, no. 1 (2005): 19–30. https://doi.org/10.1525/aa.2005.107.1.019.

TallBear, Kimberly. *Native American DNA: Tribal Belonging and the False Promise of Genetic Science*. Minneapolis: University of Minnesota Press, 2013.

Thomas, Deborah A. *Exceptional Violence: Embodied Citizenship in Transnational Jamaica*. Durham, NC: Duke University Press, 2011.

Thomas, Deborah A. *Modern Blackness: Nationalism, Globalization and the Politics of Culture in Jamaica*. Durham, NC: Duke University Press, 2004.

Thomas, Deborah A., and Kamari Maxine Clarke, eds. *Globalization and Race: Transformations in the Cultural Production of Blackness*. Durham, NC: Duke University Press, 2006.

Tinsley, O. N. "Black Atlantic, Queer Atlantic: Queer Imaginings of the Middle Passage." *GLQ: A Journal of Lesbian and Gay Studies* 14, nos. 2–3 (2008): 191–215. https://doi.org/10.1215/10642684-2007-030.

Tinsley, Omise'eke Natasha. *Thiefing Sugar: Eroticism between Women in Caribbean Literature*. Durham, NC: Duke University Press, 2010.

Tinsley, Omise'ke, Ananya Chatterjea, Hui Niu Wilcox, and Shannon Gibney. "So Much to Remind Us We Are Dancing on Other People's Blood." In *Critical Transnational Feminist Praxis*, edited by Amanda Lock Swarr and Richa Nagar, 147–65. Albany: SUNY Press, 2010.

Trostle, James A. "Medical Compliance as an Ideology." *Social Science and Medicine* 27, no. 12 (1988): 1299–308. https://doi.org/10.1016/0277-9536(88)90194-3.

Trotz, D. Alissa. "Rethinking Caribbean Transnational Connections: Conceptual Itineraries." *Global Networks* 6, no. 1 (2006): 41–59. https://doi.org/10.1111/j.1471-0374.2006.00132.x.

Trouillot, Michel-Rolph. *Global Transformations: Anthropology and the Modern World*. New York: Palgrave Macmillan, 2003.

Tuck, Eve, and K. Wayne Yang. "Decolonization Is Not a Metaphor." *Decolonization: Indigeneity, Education and Society* 1, no. 1 (2012). https://jps.library.utoronto.ca/index.php/des/article/view/18630.

United Nations Development Programme (UNDP). "Human Development Reports." UNDP, 2018. http://hdr.undp.org/en/composite/HDI.

US Central Intelligence Agency. "The World Factbook: Barbados Economy—Overview." CIA, 19 April 2016. https://www.cia.gov/library/publications/the-world-factbook/geos/bb.html.

Walcott, Corey. "Awright Den! Choose Abstinence." *Nation News*, 31 October 2013. http://www.nationnews.com/nationnews/news/2785/awright-den-choose-abstinence.

Walcott, Rinaldo. *Black Like Who? Writing Black Canada*. Toronto: Insomniac Press, 2003.

Ward, Juann M., Kolin Schmalenberg, Nick A. Antonishyn, Ian R. Hambleton, Elizabeth L. Blackman, Paul N. Levett, and Marquita V. Gittens-St.Hilaire. "Human Papillomavirus Genotype Distribution in Cervical Samples among Vaccine Naïve Barbados Women." *Cancer Causes and Control* 28, no. 11 (2017): 1323–32.

Washington, Harriet A. *Medical Apartheid: The Dark History of Medical Experimentation on Black Americans from Colonial Times to the Present*. New York: Doubleday, 2006.

Whitmarsh, Ian. *Biomedical Ambiguity: Race, Asthma, and the Contested Meaning of Genetic Research in the Caribbean*. Ithaca, NY: Cornell University Press, 2008.

Whitmarsh, Ian. "Medical Schismogenics: Compliance and 'Culture' in Caribbean Biomedicine." *Anthropological Quarterly* 82, no. 2 (2009): 447–75.

Wickham, Peter W., Carlos L. A. Wharton, Dave Marshall, and Hilda A. Darlington-Weeks. "Freedom of Movement: The Cornerstone of the Caribbean Single Market and Economy (CSME)." Caribbean Development Research Services, January 2004. https://sta.uwi.edu/salises/workshop/papers/pwickham.pdf.

Wiens, Brianna I., and Shana MacDonald. "Feminist Futures: #MeToo's Possibilities as Poiesis, Techné, and Pharmakon." *Feminist Media Studies* (1 June 2020). https://doi.org/10.1080/14680777.2020.1770312.

Wilson, Elizabeth A. *Gut Feminism*. Durham, NC: Duke University Press, 2015.

Wilson, Peter J. *Crab Antics: The Social Anthropology of English-Speaking Negro Societies of the Caribbean*. New Haven, CT: Yale University Press, 1973.

Women and Development Unit (WAND). "Demystifying and Fighting Cervical Cancer." *Women's Health Journal/Isis International* 92, no. 3 (1992): 29–51.

World Bank. "Population, Total | Data." World Bank, 2018. https://data.worldbank.org/indicator/SP.POP.TOTL?locations=BB.

World Bank. "World Development Indicators." World Bank DataBank, 2018. http://databank.worldbank.org/data/reports.aspx?source=2&country=BRB&series=&period=.

World Health Organization. "Report of the SAGE Working Group on Vaccine Hesitancy." 1 October 2014. http://www.who.int/immunization/sage/meetings/2014/october/1_Report_WORKING_GROUP_vaccine_hesitancy_final.pdf.

World Health Organization. "Vaccine Hesitancy: A Growing Challenge for Immunization Programmes." 2015. http://www.who.int/mediacentre/news/releases/2015/vaccine-hesitancy/en/.

Zachmann, Karin. "Risk in Historical Perspective: Concepts, Contexts, and Conjunctions." In *Risk—A Multidisciplinary Introduction*, edited by Claudia Klüppelberg, Daniel Straub, and Isabell M. Welpe, 3–35. Cham: Springer, 2014. https://doi.org/10.1007/978-3-319-04486-6_1.

Index

COVID-19 pandemic, 151–52, 154
creole value systems, 68–69, 169n4
criminalization, 57, 165n35

De Barros, Juanita, 163n23, 164n30
Democratic Labour Party (DLP), 9–10, 61, 157n33, 168nn55–56
Derrida, Jacques, 168n57
diseases, spread of, 16, 46, 56–58, 86, 164n30, 165n39
doctors, 40, 63, 94–95, 102, 124; authority and dismissal, 122–23, 132–33; colonial, 57, 164n30; distrust of, 98–99; suspicion and certainty of, 125–34, 139; vaccination campaigns and, 126–27

Ebola epidemic, 41, 154
economic growth, 21, 28, 30, 61, 151, 168n56
economic recession (2008), 9–10, 28, 30, 31, 38, 149
education, 9–10, 51, 61, 68, 139; community health, 140–41, 144–45, 146; sexual health, 82, 86–88, 110–11, 143; technologies for, 85; training for nurses and doctors, 126; vaccine refusal and, 76, 117–18, 123
Education Sector Enhancement Programme, 85, 170n33
elites, 55, 59, 61, 65, 166n46
embodiments, 13–14, 15, 22, 93, 107, 115; feelings, 31, 147, 149; knowledge, 110, 111; sensibilities, 6, 98–101, 106
enslaved women, 49, 55–56, 59, 163n26. See also slavery
entrepreneurship, 30–31, 43, 170n11
Epstein, Steven, 72, 81
erotic, 14, 99, 102, 107, 133, 171n6; subjugation, 16, 150
ethics, 22, 83, 137; of care, 114, 119, 147; of protection, 22, 44, 111, 113, 137, 144
eugenicist beliefs, 16, 56, 165n35
export bans, 151, 174n3

Facebook, 19, 47, 103, 115–17, 123–24, 125; HPV vaccine groups, 172n1
fake news, 119–24, 139, 152
family: lower-class Black, 57, 58–59; non-nuclear, 169n4; nuclear or normative, 68, 69, 168n53; planning, 59–60, 139, 167n50
Fanon, Frantz, 106, 145
feeling rules, 119, 132–33
femininity, 60, 72, 168n53
feminism, 168n57; health care activism, 140–41, 144; transnational, 14, 15, 18, 138, 145, 152, 159n55
feminist theorists, 7, 8, 13, 72, 114, 156n27, 159n56; affect theories, 14–15, 119, 147; mind-body theories, 102
fingerprinting, 30, 34–35
flesh theories, 14, 98, 101, 106–7, 130, 138

Food and Drug Administration (FDA), 10, 25, 157n37
force, sense of, 96–97, 100–101, 104–7, 115, 138
foreign investment, 9, 33, 35, 65, 149
Freeman, Carla, 30–31, 43, 69, 169n11, 171n39
free market, 29
free movement, 29, 31–32, 34, 161n8
futurity, 22, 101–6, 111, 113

Garcia-Rojas, Claudia, 14
Gardasil Awareness NZ, 115–17, 172nn1–2
Gardasil/Gardasil 9, 10–11, 52–53, 72, 81, 112, 127; cost, 39, 50, 125; list of reported side effects, 172n3; long-term efficacy, 128–29; promotion of, 54, 63, 74. See also side effects (of HPV vaccine)
gendered ideologies, 68–69, 76, 79, 84, 93, 109; HPV vaccine and, 71–74, 131
genetic research, 38, 161n29
genital warts, 10–11, 47, 63, 71, 108, 157n37, 163n19
Gilroy, Paul, 106
GlaxoSmithKline, 157n37
Global Alliance for Vaccines and Immunization, 156n25, 158n39
global assemblages, 84, 97, 106, 118, 121, 170n31
Global South, 140–41
Goldenberg, Maya, 120
government distrust, 10, 30, 35, 61, 82–83, 118, 149; HPV vaccine and, 36–37, 53, 76
gut feelings, 6, 94, 106, 107, 136, 138; vaccine refusal and, 27, 98–101
Guyana Chronicle (newspaper), 86
Gyn-A-Thon Barbados, 47, 48, 49, 50, 54, 63–64, 124

Hall, Stuart, 15
Harper, Diane, 128–29, 173n16
Hartman, Saidiya, 106, 147
hepatitis B vaccine, 39, 81, 127, 163n17
herbal remedies, 77, 142–44
hesitancy. See vaccine hesitancy
heteronormativity, 54, 69, 73
heteropatriarchy, 7, 69, 73–74, 92
Higginbotham, Evelyn Brooks, 167n52
Hochschild, Arlie, 119, 133
Homeland Security, US Department of, 34
homosexuality and homophobia, 36, 71–72, 92
hospitals, 49, 55, 57–58
Hottentot women, 164n35
Human Development Index (HDI), 9–10, 30, 161n11
human papillomavirus (HPV): awareness and education, 47, 48, 49, 63, 140–41; exposure to antibodies, 79; gendered disparities, 71–74; high-risk strains, 4, 47, 52–53, 102, 113; lived experiences of, 108–11; promiscuity and, 80. See also cervical cancer; genital warts

parental consent, 11, 83, 100

Paugh, Katherine, 56

Payne, Clement, 166n40

peer pressure, 87, 143

Persson, Asha, 62

pharmaceutical industry, 5, 10–11, 77, 81, 133, 160n66; financial motivations, 16, 38–41, 52, 80, 104–5; marketing and promotion, 50, 51, 109–10, 113, 149, 163n18; partnerships, 38, 84; trials and testing, 54, 64, 97–98, 131, 154

pharmaceuticalization, 76, 81, 92, 149, 151

pharmakon (term usage), 62

plantations, 56, 165n40

political activism, 166n40, 168n54, 168n57; health campaigns, 140–41, 145

polyclinics, 12, 131, 142, 159n64, 160n68, 163n19; posters at, 1, *2*, 3

postcolonial (term usage), 156n27

post-truth, 119, 139, 146, 152, 172n4

poverty, 56–57, 58, 164n30, 166n40

power: relations of, 72–73

Pranav, Heena, 3

Price, Margaret, 102

private clinics, 20, 125

privatization, 9, 28, 30

promiscuity, 57, 58, 79, 80, 131, 168n53

prostitution, 57–58, 165n36

protection, 8, 10–11, 42, 124; biomedical certainty and, 134–37; care and, 16, 17, 43, 44, 51, 114, 146; of children, 74, 76, 82; of citizens, 34, 35, 112, 122; education and, 142–43; ethics of, 22, 113, 137, 144; respectability and, 78–79, 83; sense and sensibility and, 22, 94–95, 107–8; suspicion and/as, 93, 97–98, 112–14, 117, 138; vaccine refusal and, 27, 70, 98–99, 107, 109–11, 150; of white male bodies, 57; of women's reproduction, 101–6, 108–9

Protection of Children Act, 85

psychic trauma, 98, 102, 106, 137

public clinics. *See* polyclinics

public health, 44, 56, 65, 91, 139, 150; advertisements, 1, *2*, 42, 173n14; antivaccination rhetoric and, 119–22; campaigns, 16, 19, 23, 39–40, 62, 162n10; forcefulness of, 96–97; international organizations, 39; nurses and doctors, 125–29; vaccination risks and, 46–47; vaccine hesitancy and, 5, 7, 12

racialization, 17, 23, 62, 98, 107, 121; biopolitics and, 21, 49; poor laws and, 56–57; science and, 16, 150; of sexuality, 82, 164n35; vaccine campaigns and, 63–64, 65

racism, 62, 102, 140, 166n40, 167n52; colonial

medical, 58, 152; eugenic, 59; histories of, 8, 81, 92, 106; scientific, 55, 106

radical care, 114, 147, 150–51, 154

raising awareness, 47, 49, 50, 63, 115–16, 140–41, 172n1

rationality/irrationality, 6–7, 17, 60, 114, 139, 150–51, 154; medical certainty and, 128, 130; sensibility and, 95, 98

refusal: concepts of, 12–13. *See also* vaccine refusal

reproductive technologies, 12–13, 46

resistance (term usage), 12

respectability: adolescent sexuality and, 78–80, 82, 85; Black middle-class, 60, 65, 68, 165n39, 167n52, 168n53; gendered ideologies and, 72, 74; parents' preoccupation with, 70–71, 92; politics of, 22, 67, 68–69, 75–77, 83, 90–91, 169n11; reputation and, 74; Victorian values of, 59

responsibility, 76, 82, 99–100, 111

riots, 166n40

risk: biopower/biopolitics and, 21, 46–47; Black women's sexuality and, 49, 55–60, 82; concepts and theorizations, 45–46; HPV vaccine and, 50–51, 54–55, 62–63, 163n19; masculinity and, 74; pharmaceutical assemblages and, 81, 84

Sagicor Life, 49, 162n16

sanitary conditions, 57, 112, 164n30, 165n39

Schalk, Sami, 102

schools: adolescent sexual activity in, 85–87, 89–90, 92; sanitation and security in, 112; social class and, 135, 137; vaccine delivery program, 11–12, 100, 125, 146, 158n39. *See also* education

securitization, 21, 28, 33–35

self-determination, 22–23, 55, 119, 141

self-governance, 10, 55, 60, 166n46, 168n53

sense and sensibility: biomedical, 27, 130, 137, 149; embodied, 6, 101, 106, 111, 115; of empathy, 136, 138; force and, 96–97; gut instincts, 98–99; protection and, 22, 94–95, 101–2, 107–8, 113; of suspicion, 33, 35, 38, 40, 61, 114, 145; term usage, 95

sexual health education, 82, 86–88, 110–11, 143

sexuality. *See* adolescent sexuality; Black women's sexuality; hypersexuality

sexually transmitted diseases (STDs). *See* venereal diseases

sexual modesty, 68–69, 78–80

sex work. *See* prostitution

Sheller, Mimi, 55

side effects (of HPV vaccine), 126, 129, 136–37; adverse reactions, 98–99, 134–36; disclosure of, 127, 129; Merck's list of reported, 172n3; online videos of, 115–19, 172n1; parental concerns over, 54, 70–71, 77, 79–80, 96, 100, 137; women's reproduction and, 54, 100–105 silence: around sexuality, 22, 67, 69, 71, 73, 74, 92; respectability and, 165n39, 167n52

Simpson, Audra, 13

single market economy. *See* Caribbean Single Market Economy (CSME)

slavery, 13–14, 21, 68, 92, 121; "afterlife of," 147, 152; Black flesh and, 107; epidemics and, 164n30; erotic subjugation under, 16, 150; histories of suspicion and, 81–82, 105; violence of, 91, 106, 111; women's reproduction and, 55–56, 163n26

smallpox, 46

smartphones. *See* cellphones

Smith, Faith, 69

social media, 3, 19, 88, 119, 124, 136; adolescent sexual activity and, 85–86, 89; medical disinformation and, 120–22; vaccine side effects and, 115–19, 129, 172n1. *See also* Facebook; Instagram

social norms, 68, 169n4

social partnership, 9–10, 61, 156n31, 168n56

Spillers, Hortense, 107, 172n23

spirituality, 133

Stacey, Jackie, 106

state power, 73

stereotypes, 68, 80, 153, 168n53; hypersexuality, 22, 81, 82, 165n39

sterilizations, 59, 166n46

structural adjustment policies, 9, 29, 61, 168n56

Stuart, Freundel J., 34

subjectivities, 42–43, 105, 107, 119; suspicion and certainty and, 23, 133, 138, 139

sugarcane, 9, 29

surveillance, 28, 44, 145, 153; biopolitical, 21, 50, 58, 63, 149; of Black women's bodies, 55–58, 82, 164n30

suspicion: theorizing, 12–17, 148–52

syphilis, 57, 86; Tuskegee, 98, 171n3

taboos, sex, 66, 72, 132

TallBear, Kimberly, 13

teenage pregnancy, 83

Thistlewood, Thomas, 163n26

tourism, 9, 38, 90, 151, 156n32

trade liberalization, 29

transnational communities, 118

Treaty of Chaguaramas (1973), 161n7

Trinidadians, 19, 24–25, 33, 160n66

Trouillot, Michel-Rolph, 153

Trump administration, 151, 174n3

tuberculosis vaccine, 46, 152, 162n10

Uganda, 3, 42, 173n14

United States, 6, 10, 71, 104, 119, 145; Black middle-class respectability, 68, 165n39, 167n52; export bans, 151–52, 154, 174n3

unsettling (term usage), 7–8

vaccine hesitancy: antivaccination rhetoric and fake news and, 23, 119–24; context and complexities of, 4–8; doctors' and nurses' roles in, 125–29; gendered disparities and, 70–73; "historical" tropes, 16, 149–50; parents and, 11–12, 17, 24–26, 160n67; politics of respectability and, 74–76; refusal of care and, 153–54; social media and, 115–19, 172n1; as suspicion, 12–14, 27, 43, 107, 114, 138, 145, 148; teenagers and, 66–67; term usage, 5, 27, 156n21

vaccine refusal, 3, 5, 27, 153–54, 160n67; adolescent sexuality and, 66–67, 70, 75, 79–83; distrust of government and, 36–37; doctors' and nurses' suspicions and, 128–31; education and, 76, 117–18, 123; ethical imperatives, 22; gender ideologies and, 74; gut instincts and, 98–102; pharmaceutical motives and, 41–42, 81, 82, 109–10; protection and, 109–14, 137, 149–50; public health concerns, 46, 119

vaccines. *See* Gardasil/Gardasil 9

venereal diseases, 56, 57, 86, 165n35, 165n39

Victorian values, 59, 60, 167n52

violence, 44, 145, 153, 172n20; colonial, 15, 27, 62, 64, 166n40; sexual regulation and, 57–58; slavery and, 82, 91, 105–6, 111, 163n26

virginity, 87

Wakefield, Andrew, 120, 173n8

Western behaviors, 3, 98

White affect studies, 14

whiteness, 69, 165n35

Whitmarsh, Ian, 6–7, 38–39, 161n29

Wickham, Peter, 32

Wilson, Elizabeth, 102

Wilson, Peter, 68–69

Women and Development Unit (WAND), 140–41, 145

women's health activism, 140–41

women's reproduction, 47, 49, 83; access to contraception, 83; colonial management of, 55–60, 163n26; protection and futurity of, 22, 54, 100–106, 108–9, 111, 113

working class, 59–60, 65, 165n40, 167n52; masculinity, 68, 168n53

World Bank, 29, 168n56

World Health Organization (WHO), 27, 42; SAGE Working Group, 5, 156n21

Zika virus, 42